Leon A. Pastalan
Editor

Housing Decisions for the Elderly: To Move or Not to Move

Pre-publication
REVIEWS,
COMMENTARIES,
EVALUATIONS . . .

"**M**oving or aging in place seems to be one of the most difficult dilemmas for older Americans within the context of their lives and their living conditions. This insightful volume thoroughly explores the crucial decisions many elderly face and provides a comprehensive overview of the complex problems that are associated with these decisions. The scope of the study papers harbors significant implications for housing America's elderly."

Benyamin Schwarz, PhD
Assistant Professor,
Environmental Design Department,
University of Missouri

More pre-publication
REVIEWS, COMMENTARIES, EVALUATIONS . . .

"Researchers, sociologists, policy makers, practitioners, builder-developers and marketing organizations of elderly housing could all benefit from reading "Housing Decisions for the Elderly: To Move or Not to Move," edited by Dr. Leon Pastalan. There is something of value for each group, offering a depth of understanding of diverse factors including, among others, the socioeconomic determinants of the housing decisions of elderly homeowners, decisions to move to a continuing care retirement community, information needs and sources for selecting senior housing and home builder attitudes and knowledge of aging and consequent relationship to design for independent living.

The papers are well researched and together provide an excellent source for review and understanding of the complex decision-making process seniors face in considering a move from their present home. As the demographics indicate, the number of persons living longer and consequently, considering a move, is increasing rapidly. Dr. Pastalan in his overview states "The variety of living arrangements is very extensive and it behooves us to be aware of this diversity and complexity."

Helen Naimark, MSW
Specialist in Aging

"The growth in the number of older households has prompted developers to invest millions of dollars in a variety of housing options intended to entice members of the potential older market to overcome their strong natural preference to stay put.

It is my impression that the planning of housing for the senior market has suffered from inadequate understanding of what actually drives the housing decisions of older households. This book addresses this weakness by bringing together the work of scholars from a variety of perspectives who address why and how the seniors themselves go about making housing decisions. The questions asked are different than those asked in a typical marketing or demographic study and they yield a number of insights that should be of value to developers and to social planners as well."

John Merrill, D. Arch
Professor and Extension Housing Specialist,
University of Wisconsin-Madison

The Haworth Press, Inc.

Housing Decisions for the Elderly: To Move or Not to Move

Housing Decisions for the Elderly: To Move or Not to Move

Leon A. Pastalan
Editor

The Haworth Press, Inc.
New York • London

Housing Decisions for the Elderly: To Move or Not to Move has also been published as *Journal of Housing for the Elderly*, Volume 11, Number 2 1995.

The Haworth Press, Inc., 10 Alice Street, Binghamton, NY 13904-1580 USA

Library of Congress Cataloging-in-Publication Data

Housing decisions for the elderly : to move or not to move / Leon A. Pastalan, editor.
    p. cm.
    Includes bibliographical references.
    ISBN 1-56024-713-4 (alk. paper)
    1. Aged–Housing–United States. 2. Old age assistance–United States. I. Pastalan, Leon A., 1930- .
HD7287.92.U5H677 1995
363.5'946'0973–dc20

95-22642
CIP

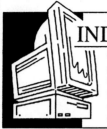

INDEXING & ABSTRACTING

Contributions to this publication are selectively indexed or abstracted in print, electronic, online, or CD-ROM version(s) of the reference tools and information services listed below. This list is current as of the copyright date of this publication. See the end of this section for additional notes.

- *Abstracts in Social Gerontology: Current Literature on Aging*, National Council on the Aging, Library, 409 Third Street SW, 2nd Floor, Washington, DC 20024

- *AgeLine Database*, American Association of Retired Persons, 601 E Street, NW, Washington, DC 20049

- *AGRICOLA Database*, National Agricultural Library, 10301 Baltimore Boulevard, Room 002, Beltsville, MD 20705

- *Applied Social Sciences Index & Abstracts (ASSIA) (Online: ASSI via Data-Star) (CDRom: ASSIA Plus)*, Bowker-Saur Limited, Maypole House, Maypole Road, East Grinstead, West Sussex RH19 1HH, England

- *Architectural Periodicals Index*, The British Architectural Library, RIBA, 66 Portland Place, London W1N 4AD, England

- *Communication Abstracts*, Temple University, 303 Annenberg Hall, Philadelphia, PA 19122

- *GEO Abstracts (GEO Abstracts/GEOBASE)*, Elsevier/GEO Abstracts, Regency House, 34 Duke Street, Norwich NR3 3AP, England

- *Human Resources Abstracts (HRA)*, Sage Publications, Inc., 2455 Teller Road, Newbury Park, CA 91320

(continued)

- *INTERNET ACCESS (& additional networks) Bulletin Board for Libraries ("BUBL"), coverage of information resources on INTERNET, JANET, and other networks.*
  - JANET X.29: UK.AC.BATH.BUBL or 00006012101300
  - TELNET: BUBL.BATH.AC.UK or 138.38.32.45 login 'bubl'
  - Gopher: BUBL.BATH.AC.UK (138.32.32.45). Port 7070
  - World Wide Web: http: / / www.bubl.bath.ac.uk./BUBL/ home.html
  - NISSWAIS: telnetniss.ac.uk (for the NISS gateway)
  The Andersonian Library, Curran Building, 101 St. James Road, Glasgow G4 ONS, Scotland

- *Inventory of Marriage and Family Literature (online and hard copy)*, National Council on Family Relations, 3989 Central Avenue NE, Suite 550, Minneapolis, MN 55421

- *Journal of Planning Literature*, Ohio State University-Department of City & Regional Planning, 190 West 17th Avenue, Columbus, OH 43210

- *Mental Health Abstracts (online through DIALOG)*, IFI/Plenum Data Company, 3202 Kirkwood Highway, Wilmington, DE 19808

- *National Library Database on Homelessness*, National Coalition for the Homeless, 1612 K Street, NW, #1004, Homelessness Information Exchange, Washington, DC 20006

- *OT BibSys*, American Occupational Therapy Foundation, P.O. Box 31220, Rockville, MD 20824-1220

- *Public Affairs Information Bulletin (PAIS)*, Public Affairs Information Service, Inc., 521 West 43rd Street, New York, NY 10036-4396

- *Sage Urban Studies Abstracts (SUSA)*, Sage Publications, Inc., 2455 Teller Road, Newbury Park, CA 91320

- *Social Planning/Policy & Development Abstracts (SOPODA)*, Sociological Abstracts, Inc., P.O. Box 22206, San Diego, CA 92192-0206

(continued)

- *Sociological Abstracts (SA)*, Sociological Abstracts, Inc.,
  P.O. Box 22206, San Diego, CA 92192-0206

- *Urban Affairs Abstracts*, National League of Cities,
  1301 Pennsylvania Avenue NW, Washington, DC 20004

SPECIAL BIBLIOGRAPHIC NOTES

*related to special journal issues (separates)
and indexing/abstracting*

☐ indexing/abstracting services in this list will also cover material in any "separate" that is co-published simultaneously with Haworth's special thematic journal issue or DocuSerial. Indexing/abstracting usually covers material at the article/chapter level.

☐ monographic co-editions are intended for either non-subscribers or libraries which intend to purchase a second copy for their circulating collections.

☐ monographic co-editions are reported to all jobbers/wholesalers/approval plans. The source journal is listed as the "series" to assist the prevention of duplicate purchasing in the same manner utilized for books-in-series.

☐ to facilitate user/access services all indexing/abstracting services are encouraged to utilize the co-indexing entry note indicated at the bottom of the first page of each article/chapter/contribution.

☐ this is intended to assist a library user of any reference tool (whether print, electronic, online, or CD-ROM) to locate the monographic version if the library has purchased this version but not a subscription to the source journal.

☐ individual articles/chapters in any Haworth publication are also available through the Haworth Document Delivery Services (HDDS).

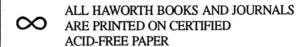

Housing Decisions for the Elderly: To Move or Not to Move

CONTENTS

ABOUT THE EDITOR

Leon A. Pastalan, PhD, is Professor of Architecture in the College of Architecture and Urban Planning at the University of Michigan. Dr. Pastalan is also Director of the National Center on Housing and Living Arrangements for Older Americans. As a researcher of long standing in the field of environments for the elderly, he is an expert in sensory deficits, spatial behavior, and housing. Dr. Pastalan has published many books and articles resulting from his work, including *Man Environment Reference 2 (MER 2)*, (The University of Michigan Press, 1983), *Retirement Communities: An American Original* (The Haworth Press, Inc., 1984), *Lifestyles and Housing of Older Adults: The Florida Experience* (The Haworth Press, Inc., 1989), *Aging in Place: The Role of Housing and Social Supports* (The Haworth Press, Inc., 1990), and *Optimizing Housing for the Elderly: Homes Not Houses* (The Haworth Press, Inc., 1991). Dr. Pastalan is also Editor of the *Journal of Housing for the Elderly* (The Haworth Press, Inc.).

Chapter 1

Overview

Leon A. Pastalan

To move or not to move is really part of the aging in place debate. While most people wish to age in place, these same people give little time to the consideration of future housing options. There is some evidence which suggests that people who move, particularly those who move from a cold climate to a warm climate are different from those who don't make such moves. These persons tend to have a higher socioeconomic status and may in fact have more than one residence throughout a given year.

The variety of living arrangements are very extensive and it behooves us to be aware of this diversity and complexity. We know for instance that approximately 80% of elderly men live in family settings but only about one-half of older women do.

It is also important to point out that the proportion living in a family setting decreases with age, so that the older the person, the more likely he or she will be living alone or with non-relatives. There are increasing numbers of elderly persons who are faced with sharp and drastic cuts in disposable income upon retirement. The problem of low income is frequently compounded by health problems. Changes in household composition typically occur at one or more points in the aging process, for example, when a spouse dies or suffers an incapacitating illness, alternative housing solutions must be found. These changes in marital and health status tend to

[Haworth co-indexing entry note]: "Overview." Pastalan, Leon A. Co-published simultaneously in *Journal of Housing for the Elderly* (The Haworth Press, Inc.) Vol. 11, No. 2, 1995, pp. 1-4; and: *Housing Decisions for the Elderly: To Move or Not to Move* (ed: Leon A. Pastalan) The Haworth Press, Inc., 1995, pp. 1-4. Multiple copies of this article/chapter may be purchased from The Haworth Document Delivery Center [1-800-3-HAWORTH; 9:00 a.m. - 5:00 p.m. (EST)].

make remaining in one's residence increasingly more difficult. The net result may be a reduction in choice of moving or not moving.

It is important to remember that the retirement period may last for a very long time and the changes in economic circumstances, household composition and health, place a great deal of pressure on these households and frequently leads them to alter their housing situation several times between the onset of retirement and death.

Housing decisions in terms of moving or not moving are one of life's most difficult decisions. Difficult because it fundamentally impacts on every facet of life. In addition to the important concerns discussed above, one's home has a psychological and metaphysical significance over and above being a shelter in which to conduct everyday life. It is a place of protection, a refuge; it also has symbolic properties that give a place meaning and significance. Spatial and environmental settings support patterns of experience and behavior. Activities such as dining, visiting, watching television, cleaning, sleeping, etc., help to orient us in space, time, and sociocultural context. These elements by their daily presence serve to remind us of who we are. It is a tangible relationship between people and the places where we dwell.

Is it any wonder that people, particularly elderly people have such reluctance to move. VanderHart correctly points out that much of the research dealing with the subject focuses primarily on mobility issues and thus sheds little light on other determinants of housing change. His research suggests a number of factors which have significant effects on decisions to move such as housing characteristics, length of tenure, gender, age and support from relatives. Guidry and Shilling also feel that demographic characteristics, particularly age, impact significantly on whether an older person owns or rents. Renting for example may be appropriate for someone who has an alternative need or use for the money that would otherwise be tied up as equity in a home. Owning, on the other hand, often ties down the shelter costs for elderly households and provides them with greater choices to better satisfy their space needs. Morgan and Krach focused their research on what kind of information consumers and professionals want to know. They found that many consumers do not have a clear idea of where to turn for information on housing. They also discovered that cost and services are the most central issues to consumers, while professionals focus on functional impairment and space availability. Liebig found a specific professional group, State Units on Aging and Housing for the Elderly, whose activity in housing has been in the area of service coordination and that housing has not been a high priority. She concluded that this organization must redefine housing as part of community based care, and expand their capacity building and expertise in housing by resetting priorities and reallocating budgets in order to better serve the older consumer.

Johnson-Carroll, Brandt and McFadden studied the relative contributions of factors influencing preference to move on retirement. They report that years in the community, tenure preference upon retirement, opinion of size of house suitable for retirement and existence of plans on where to retire led to preference and propensity to move. Sheehan and Karasik studied a newly opened continuing care retirement community and found that residents evidenced significantly more "risk" factors than waiting list applicants and reported significantly more reasons for selecting a CCRC. Reasons for choosing a CCRC included guaranteed access to health care, freedom from home maintenance, and supportive services. Belser and Weber examined the relationship between home builders' attitudes and knowledge of aging and their awareness and use of accessible products and architectural features in residential design. Results indicated that home builders tended to think somewhat negatively about the elderly and were aware of more accessible products and design features than they actually used. The majority of builders reported that accessible product and design features in a residence was a viable idea but their use depended on client awareness and request. Finally VanderHart presents a model of housing decision making of elderly homeowners that represents perhaps the first attempt to integrate multiple elements impacting on housing decisions into a single framework. While the model is highly theoretical and has a number of shortcomings, it does suggest how a large number of decisional factors having differential effects across various housing changes may be organized for analysis and therefore have an eventual impact on housing policy and practice.

This publication has identified a number of significant factors regarding decisions to move which have important implications for policy makers, developers and marketers, academics, housing professionals and others concerned with why elderly people move or do not move.

There remains an entire domain of inquiry which has not received attention in the literature that deals specifically with symbolic aspects of moving out of one's home such as personal identity, privacy, control, family history and the like. The place we call home evokes an image of affection, loyalty, obligations and responsibilities. There appears to be no question that this important domain needs to be addressed by those of us in the housing field.

Chapter 2

The Socioeconomic Determinants of the Housing Decisions of Elderly Homeowners

Peter G. VanderHart

SUMMARY. Evidence suggests that demographic considerations may be more important than financial considerations to elderly homeowners' housing decisions. Cross-tabulations on marital, employment, children, and disability factors yield strong, intuitively consistent results as to their effect on housing changes. Financial variables, on the other hand, have less consistent results. Home equity and housing costs do not have consistently strong relationships across housing transitions. Where they do have relationships, they are often different from what is indicated by intuition. The results for income and financial assets are somewhat better, but are not particularly strong. Overall these results suggest that demographic factors are much more important than financial factors in elderly homeowners' housing decisions.

Decisions regarding housing are among the most dramatic that elderly homeowners make. A home is usually the household's larg-

Peter G. VanderHart is Assistant Professor of Economics, Department of Economics, Bowling Green State University, Bowling Green, OH 43403-0268.

[Haworth co-indexing entry note]: "The Socioeconomic Determinants of the Housing Decisions of Elderly Homeowners." VanderHart, Peter G. Co-published simultaneously in *Journal of Housing for the Elderly* (The Haworth Press, Inc.) Vol. 11, No. 2, 1995, pp. 5-35; and: *Housing Decisions for the Elderly: To Move or Not to Move* (ed: Leon A. Pastalan) The Haworth Press, Inc., 1995, pp. 5-35. Multiple copies of this article/chapter may be purchased from The Haworth Document Delivery Center [1-800-3-HAWORTH; 9:00 a.m. - 5:00 p.m. (EST)].

est consumer durable and the largest portion of its investment port-folio. A home also usually represents much more than an asset and a source of consumption services. A certain degree of status and a sense of independence comes with home ownership, and it may be a source of many memories. A housing change represents a drastic change in these dimensions, and the move from one's home may involve considerable disruption, which may be of particular con-cern for the elderly.

Several government programs have an impact on the elderly's choice of living arrangement. Some of these seem designed to help the elderly remain homeowners (such as heating subsidies and property tax deduction and deferment programs, or the fact that home equity is not usually included as an asset for welfare program qualification purposes), while others seem to encourage movement out of owner-occupied housing (the exemption of $125,000 in capi-tal gains on housing and the different reimbursement policies ap-plied to institutional versus in-home health care). There has also been some discussion about the potential of reverse mortgages and similar instruments to allow the elderly to tap their home equity (Jacobs, 1986; Scholen and Chen, 1981).

Despite the importance of understanding these decisions to both public and private concerns, it appears that the process is not com-pletely understood. To date research has not examined all the hous-ing changes that the elderly make, and has been unable to clearly identify what considerations are most important in the elderly's housing decisions. Specifically, the research tends to concentrate only on mobility, and thus does not distinguish between different types of housing changes. It also has been unable to determine whether financial or demographic factors are the more important determinants of the decision. This paper seeks to shed some light on the topic.

The paper is organized as follows: The next section describes the various housing changes available to an elderly homeowner, and discusses some of the frequently mentioned causal factors of the changes. Later sections describe the data used in this article and present new evidence regarding these issues. The final sections summarize the results, discuss their policy implications, and sug-gest future work.

DESCRIPTIONS AND DETERMINANTS OF THE HOUSING CHOICES AVAILABLE TO ELDERLY HOMEOWNERS

Potential Housing Changes by Elderly Homeowners

The economic theories known as the life-cycle and permanent income hypotheses (see Stoller and Stoller, 1987) imply that households will draw upon their assets to finance consumption later in life. Given that owner-occupied housing often makes up such a large portion of the elderly's assets, it is not unreasonable to think that they may wish to reduce the amount of this asset in some way to increase consumption.

One way to enable dissaving out of home equity would be for the household to acquire a reverse mortgage. This instrument provides a flow of income without subjecting the household to moving costs. However, Manchester (1987) has observed that households with low incomes also tend to have low home equity, so low that a reverse mortgage would not provide substantial additional income to people who need it the most. In addition, the market for reverse mortgages was practically non-existent until a short time ago. Only about 100 had been written by 1984 (Weinrobe, 1984), and only in the last few years have private financial companies begun to offer reverse mortgages on a nationwide basis (PHIP, 1989).

If a reverse mortgage is unavailable or not desirable, some households may want to acquire a conventional mortgage or home equity loan to utilize their accumulated home equity. This action may be ill-suited for many elderly households because of the initial cost of any mortgage and the interest rate difference between a mortgage and the investment of its proceeds. Of course the acquisition of a mortgage does not necessarily entail a decrease in home equity: If the proceeds are used to remodel or improve the home, the equity of the home could increase. Also, although acquiring a mortgage may initially be an act of dissaving, it forces the household to save as the mortgage payments are made.

If an elderly household decides that acquiring a reverse or conventional mortgage is not an alternative, it may decide to move to a home with lower equity or move into a rental unit. These sorts of moves would also allow the household to utilize its home equity to increase consumption. Although they would subject the household to the financial and psychological costs of moving, actions such as these could also allow the elderly to cut their housing expenditures, and the potentially smaller size of the new unit could be easier to maintain.

The homeowner may also find for various reasons that movement into a dependent living arrangement is desired. This might include living with children or with others, entering a nursing home or assisted-living community, or having one's housing paid for by others. These sorts of moves may also allow the household to increase consumption by drawing down home equity, but it is unclear whether the dependent elderly are able to enjoy the extra consumption.

Some homeowners may not want to reduce their home equity and may actually wish to increase it: Some of the elderly increase their home equity by moving to a more expensive home. This sort of move is not necessarily at odds with economic models of consumption during old age: Households may dissave only out of other assets, or a home may play a special role as a bequest.

All of these housing changes may occur for reasons unrelated to the inherent financial considerations. Older households may find that a large home is difficult to maintain and is not needed once children have moved away, and in the process of moving to a smaller home they will likely reduce their home equity. The onset of disability or widowhood may make non-owning alternatives attractive (for reasons other than purely financial ones), and this entails a complete liquidation of home equity. For these reasons, any analysis examining housing changes should include both financial *and* demographic considerations.

Factors Affecting the Homeowner's Decision

Here we discuss the factors frequently mentioned as the major determinants of elderly homeowners' housing decisions. After the discussion we briefly describe some results of past empirical studies. We begin by describing financial factors, and move on to demographic considerations.

Home Equity. Intuitively, one should expect high levels of home equity to cause an increased desire to undertake a housing change that reduces home equity: The more home equity a household has, the more useful its proceeds would be as a way to pay for unexpected expenses or to supplement a fixed income.

Financial Assets. Households with greater amounts of non-housing assets are likely to be less prone to reducing their home equity. Wealthier households are better able to dissave out of their liquid assets to enhance consumption or pay for an unexpected expense. This allows them to avoid the transaction costs associated with reducing home equity, and still enjoy the benefits that home ownership provides. Note that this implies that high levels of financial assets will deter moves that reduce home equity, while high levels of home equity will promote such moves. Any rigorous treatment will therefore treat home equity and financial assets separately.

Income. For the most part, income should have an effect similar to that of financial assets: The more income a household has, the less it needs to dissave out of any asset (including home equity) to finance additional consumption or pay for unexpected expenses. However, higher levels of income may also enable older households to afford the monetary costs of moving, thus making housing change more likely.

The Out-of-Pocket Cost of Housing. Many elderly households own their home outright, or have relatively small mortgage payments on a favorable mortgage written long ago. Yet they must still make property tax payments, and provide for their home's maintenance. This may be difficult if the household is on a fixed income and the home's assessed value is large, maintenance costs are large or frequent, or the owners are unable to perform routine maintenance themselves. It is expected that high housing expenses will cause elderly homeowners to take actions that reduce home equity. (Of course high home ownership costs will only drive homeowners out of their house if a cheaper alternative is available.)

Employment Status. We now turn our attention to determinants that are not measured in dollar terms, and can be considered more demographic in nature. We begin with a factor closely related to the financial factors, employment status. The onset of retirement may be an important cause of elderly homeowners deciding to leave their homes. The retirement years are often the time where the elderly move to warm climates and retirement-oriented communities. Not having a job reduces the costs of a location change, and the date of retirement may mark the beginning of the household's desire to dissave, possibly out of home equity.

Physical Limitation. Physical limitation and bad health may have an adverse effect on a homeowner's ability to maintain a house. A limitation can make some maintenance activities difficult, and could force the elderly to have maintenance done by more expensive outside help. Limitations may also affect the homeowner's ability to perform everyday tasks in an independent living situation, thus causing a move to a dependent arrangement. Liquidated home equity could be used to pay medical bills or to finance in-home care. If physically limited elderly homeowners have no children nearby and are financially constrained, one would expect them to be more prone to leave their home for an assisted-living arrangement.

Familial Considerations. The presence of a spouse or children may increase the attachment that a household has for a home. Married homeowners may have a special psychological attachment to the home in which they have both lived. Each of the family members will experience disruption if a housing change is made, making a move for couples more costly in psychological terms. An older couple may also be better able to maintain a home than a single person. The onset of widowhood often entails a drop in income and possibly an increase in expenses, and this could make the liquidation of home equity attractive.

Children who live with their elderly parents can also help with maintenance, and add to the family's disruption if they move. Even if the elderly's children do not live with them, their presence in the area may cause their parents to hold on to a home longer than otherwise. Independent children may be able to aid in the maintenance of the home, or care for the elderly in the home during short illnesses. Danziger, Schwartz, and Smolensky (1984) have suggested that elderly parents may hold homes of excess size as a form of insurance for their children, to be used as a refuge during spells of financial difficulty. The elderly's home may also be viewed as the center of an extended family, where they can meet for holidays and special occasions. The home may also play a special role in the elderly's bequest motive.

Previous Work

Financial Factors. Several articles examine the effect of various financial factors on the home ownership decisions of the elderly. There appears to be no consensus among the articles about the effect of financial assets and home equity (Merrill, 1984; Feinstein and McFadden, 1987; Venti and Wise, 1989, 1990; Reschovsky, 1990). Further mixed evidence is present with regards to the effect of income, although generally it appears that higher levels of income encourage home ownership and deter movements into dependent living arrangements (Boersch-Supan, 1989; Boersch-Supan, Kotlikoff, and Morris, 1989; Boersch-Supan, Hajivassiliou, Kotlikoff, and Morris, 1990; Ellwood and Kane, 1989; Garber and MaCurdy, 1989). Although gerontological work links high housing costs with homeowner dissatisfaction (O'Bryant and Wolf, 1982), other work appears to dispute this notion (Venti and Wise, 1989; Ai, Feinstein, McFadden, and Pollakowski, 1990).

There are a number of reasons to criticize this previous evidence. Much of the work concentrates merely on mobility, thus obscuring the underlying changes in tenure and amount of home equity. While our discussion suggests that home equity and financial assets may have different effects, several of the articles combine them into a single variable. Also, in general the transition from home ownership to dependency has not been isolated from all types of moves to dependency.

Demographic Factors. These articles and others also examine the effect of some demographic factors. Several authors have observed that being and becoming retired is correlated with housing changes (Venti and Wise, 1989; Feinstein and McFadden, 1987). Other works examine health factors, and find that deteriorating health has little effect on changes where the household stays independent, but seems to precipitate moves into nursing homes and other dependent arrangements (Merrill, 1984; Venti and Wise, 1989; Garber and MaCurdy, 1989; Ellwood and Kane, 1989; Kotlikoff and Morris, 1988).

There are many articles that examine the role of marital status on the elderly's housing changes. This literature indicates that being single or becoming a widow often tends to precipitate housing changes (Reschovsky, 1990; Feinstein and McFadden, 1987; Venti and Wise, 1989), especially moves into dependent arrangements (Garber and MaCurdy, 1989; Ellwood and Kane, 1989; Boersch-Supan 1989; Kotlikoff and Morris, 1988). The presence of children in the household also seems to have an effect on the elderly's housing decisions, with the presence of children reducing both mobility and the likelihood that an owner becomes a renter (Venti and Wise, 1990; Feinstein and McFadden, 1987).

These articles suggest that the housing decisions of elderly homeowners are complicated and involve many factors. Unfortunately, no single article examines all the factors discussed here, making it difficult to make comparisons regarding the relative importance of the various factors. They often aggregate their financial variables unnecessarily, which confuses their interpretation. Finally, the articles often focus only on mobility, and thus do not distinguish very different housing changes from one another. Therefore factors may appear to be weak because they have dramatic effects on one type of housing change and no effect on another. These shortcomings are remedied below where we examine a number of factors' effects on several possible housing changes.

DATA

Data Set Selection

The empirical study of the home ownership decisions of the elderly requires that we have data containing a large panel of older households with sufficient information on housing, financial, and demographic variables. Three sets of data were considered: The Annual Housing Survey (AHS), the Retirement History Survey (RHS), and the Panel Study of Income Dynamics (PSID). The AHS, with its panel of houses rather than occupants, lacks information on the destination of the occupants that move from their houses. Although the RHS is superior to the PSID in measuring financial assets, the RHS only has biennial observations, and lasts only ten years. Additionally, the oldest original respondent in the last wave of the RHS is 73 years old, which omits housing changes by the very old. The PSID has no such age limit, has yearly observations, and currently has 20 years of information available. These factors make the PSID the most attractive.

Structure and Relevant Variables in the PSID

The PSID began in 1968 with information on 18,230 individuals in 4,802 families. Over the 20-year history of the PSID, data has been collected on 37,530 individuals. Although it is not a panel of the elderly per se, it does contain a large number of older respondents. Over 1,400 of the original households had heads over 50 years of age in the first year of the panel. The PSID's individual-level data contain a record for each sample member. Household-level data can be obtained by selecting one individual from each household. The analyses in this work utilize such data and combine data from two adjacent years to define housing changes.

Housing Variables. The housing variables contained in the PSID are quite adequate. In each of the twenty waves respondents are asked whether they own, rent, or have other living arrangements. If they have other arrangements they are asked whether housing is some form of payment for services, is paid for by others, has been sold but not vacated, is temporary quarters, or if they will inherit the housing at a later date. In all of the waves since '68, the household is asked whether they moved during the past year. If the household does own the home, its value is recorded in all years. In most years mortgage information (amount of remaining principle, mortgage payment, number of years remaining) is recorded, the exceptions being '68, '73-'75, and '82. In addition to annual mortgage payment, measures of some of the other housing costs are available in most years: Annual utility payments for '68-'72 and '77-'87; property tax paid in all years except '78; and for renters, annual rental payments in all years.

Income and Asset Variables. As its name implies, the PSID has excellent data on respondents' income. Although close to being complete, the income data are not perfect. Taxable income is available in every year, but transfer income is not included in the first wave. Head's asset income and financial help from relatives are available only as bracket variables for '68-'75. Wife's asset income is also bracketed over this period, except that it is not recorded in the first two years of the survey.

Data on asset levels are probably the PSID's biggest weakness. Except for one year (1984) data on asset levels are not recorded. Qualitative questions about the households' savings are only asked intermittently in the early waves and not all asset types are included. Thus we must use asset income to impute households' asset level as explained below.

Demographic Variables. The demographic variables contained in the PSID are quite satisfactory. Employment status is available in each year, with responses in this category as follows: Working, temporarily laid off, unemployed, retired, permanently or temporarily disabled, keeping house, student, and other. A subjective indicator of head's disability is present in all waves but the first. In each year marital status of head is recorded, with potential responses being married or permanently cohabiting, single, widowed, divorced, or separated. The number of children present in the household is also recorded in each year.

Sample Selection, Idiosyncrasies, and Special Procedures

Sample Selection and Headship Idiosyncrasies. Because we are interested in analyzing housing decisions at the household level, use of the full individual-level panel is inappropriate because many households will contain more than one elderly individual. Because the PSID defines most of its data according to who is considered the head of household, (for instance, all members of a particular family will have identical values for "age of head" and "taxable income of head"), we select the head to provide the data that represents the household.

Because we concentrate on housing changes, the household's data must be consistent from one year to the next. A problem could arise if the person designated as head is not the same year to year. Fortunately the PSID is very consistent as to whom they define as head one year to the next. Once a respondent is designated head of household they will remain so until they die or become a nonrespondent. The PSID is also rather sexist in headship definition: In married households the male is always designated the head unless he is incapable of answering the questions.

The PSID is somewhat strange in that it gives headship status to both a husband who is newly deceased or has moved out, *and* the wife who takes over as head in the year immediately after the husband's exit. Fortunately the survey also records a "sequence number" which always has a value of one for the current head and higher values for family members who have moved out or are newly deceased. Selecting respondents based on their sequence number in the second of the two adjacent years then eliminates the possibility that the same household will be measured twice in our sample.

Households in which a wife takes over as head due to the husband's death are of some concern. Housing changes may be more likely to occur in these circumstances as a result of the change in family composition. Yet if we define a household only as those with the same head in each year we will exclude this sort of household and possibly mask important housing changes. We therefore make a point of including wives that take over as heads in the analyses. This requires some data manipulation that involves the substitution of the wife's data in place of the deceased husband's. Fortunately enough "wife" and individual-level variables are present to accomplish this. The only shortcoming is that wife's disability status is unavailable in '68, '73-'75, '79, and '80. In the analysis that uses this variable, wives that become heads in these years are excluded.

Housing Status Peculiarities. In the previous section, we described the variable that records whether the household owns, rents, or has some other living arrangement. For most respondents this variable is accurate, but for a small number of the dependent elderly it is not. Specifically, some of the elderly who live dependently with relatives are mistakenly given their relative's housing status. These persons are reclassified using a procedure similar to the one developed by the PSID staff in conjunction with David Ellwood and Thomas Kane (1989): We classify respondents as "dependent sharers" if they are single, move in with relatives, and their income remains less than half of the total family income for at least three years after the move or until they move out.

Another housing change that is not well-defined by the PSID is movement into a nursing home. The survey contains an indicator of nonresponse due to institutionalization, but this is of little use when classifying current respondents. Only in the last four waves is there a nursing home indicator for current respondents. To classify nursing home residents in earlier years we backcode from the earliest wave that the indicator is present, and rely on another procedure developed by Ellwood and Kane (1989): If the respondent moves for involuntary reasons into housing that has less than 3 rooms and reports that she neither owns nor rents, we classify her as being in a nursing home.

Weights. In its first year, the PSID oversampled the poor and nonwhites because of interest in the special role they play in income dynamics. It also clustered its sample geographically to reduce collection costs. Therefore the PSID staff provides weights for each individual in each year that can be used to adjust for the oversampling. The weights are proportional to the inverse of the probability of selection from the universe of all households in the 48 contiguous states. Over the years of the study the weights have been adjusted to account for family composition changes and differential nonresponse (see PSID's User Guide [1973] for a thorough discussion).

EMPIRICAL RESULTS

This section describes some empirical results on housing transitions of elderly homeowners. We begin by examining mobility rates, and of those that move, their tenure choice. We then concentrate on the propensity of elderly homeowners to make various housing changes. Crosstabulations of these changes by demographic and financial characteristics are presented.

The observations are defined using variables from two adjacent years. Sample members must be fifty years of age or older in the initial wave of the survey, they must be a head or wife in the first of the two adjacent years, and have a sequence number equal to one in the second. Observations are then pooled over the twenty years of the panel, which allows nineteen possible cross sections to be observed and pooled together.

Mobility Rates

Table 1 presents weighted mobility rates by age bracket. The sample is divided into 3 groups representing the different tenure classifications in the initial year. The rates differ across previous

TABLE 1. Weighted Annual Mobility Rates Within Age Group and Prior Year's Tenure Status

	Owners	Renters	Others
Age Group			
50-54	4.50% (706)	20.66% (484)	32.89% (71)
55-59	5.74% (1699)	17.66% (1012)	18.01% (134)
60-64	4.61% (2656)	14.99% (1267)	27.30% (196)
65-69	3.87% (3098)	13.86% (1217)	22.72% (214)
70-74	3.78% (2530)	10.81% (922)	16.01% (183)
75-79	4.82% (1674)	12.96% (551)	10.21% (134)
80-84	6.00% (901)	9.95% (300)	12.76% (105)
85+	8.36% (453)	13.50% (170)	9.04% (86)
All Groups	4.68% (13717)	13.71% (5923)	17.24% (1123)

Note: Numbers in parentheses represent actual unweighted numbers in each category.

tenure status, with renters and those neither owning nor renting (others) having much higher rates than owners. A chi square test (2 degrees of freedom, 1% level) rejects the hypothesis that the aggregate mobility rates do not differ across previous tenure. ($\chi^2 = 674.8$).

Within the owning group, mobility rates form a bowl shape with respect to age, with the minimum occurring when homeowners are in their early 70's. A chi-square test rejects the hypothesis that owners' mobility rates are the same across age brackets (7 degrees of freedom, 1% level, $\chi^2 = 29.9$). A possible explanation for the U-shaped rates is that owners may make housing adjustments when relatively young in response to job and family changes; and when relatively old due to deteriorating health.

Tenure Transition Matrices

Mere mobility rates tell us little about the destination tenure of those households that move, and thus omit valuable information. To remedy this we present a tenure transition matrix (similar to that in Feinstein and McFadden, 1987) in Table 2. It specifies the proportion of moving households in each initial tenure group that switches into each post-move tenure group. Table 2 provides evidence that a modest net movement away from home ownership occurs among the elderly. The movement occurs in spite of the fact that non-owners tend to be more mobile.

To explore this aspect further we present the analogous matrices for various age groups in Table 3. If we concentrate on the rows describing homeowners we see that movement into "other" tenure arrangements generally increases with age. Also, movement from home ownership to rental units is relatively high for the youngest age examined, is low for those in their early 60's, and generally rises with age thereafter. This observation is confirmed by a chi-square test involving owners only: The hypothesis that the owners'

TABLE 2. Weighted Tenure Transition Matrix for All Movers

		New Tenure		
		Own	Rent	Other
	Own	.584 (359)	.288 (188)	.128 (86)
Initial Tenure	Rent	.181 (127)	.713 (672)	.106 (82)
	Other	.286 (48)	.369 (85)	.345 (75)

Note: Numbers in parentheses are unweighted cell counts. They do not yield the percentages due to weighting.

TABLE 3. Weighted Tenure Transition Matrices Within Age Group

New Tenure

		Own	Rent	Other
	Own	.625 (78)	.326 (43)	.048 (11)
Initial Tenure	Rent	.259 (51)	.690 (210)	.050 (17)
	Other	.397 (15)	.224 (13)	.379 (20)

Age (50-59)

New Tenure

		Own	Rent	Other
	Own	.793 (85)	.139 (24)	.068 (8)
Initial Tenure	Rent	.270 (36)	.633 (137)	.097 (12)
	Other	.249 (8)	.429 (25)	.323 (13)

Age (60-64)

New Tenure

		Own	Rent	Other
	Own	.659 (74)	.231 (26)	.111 (16)
Initial Tenure	Rent	.221 (23)	.649 (133)	.130 (21)
	Other	.300 (8)	.346 (18)	.354 (18)

Age (65-69)

TABLE 3 (continued)

New Tenure

		Own	Rent	Other
	Own	.577 (53)	.320 (32)	.102 (11)
Initial Tenure	Rent	.092 (7)	.802 (87)	.106 (12)
	Other	.174 (5)	.527 (15)	.300 (11)

Age (70-74)

New Tenure

		Own	Rent	Other
	Own	.333 (28)	.439 (35)	.228 (20)
Initial Tenure	Rent	.115 (8)	.782 (60)	.103 (8)
	Other	.508 (8)	.162 (4)	.331 (5)

Age (75-80)

New Tenure

		Own	Rent	Other
	Own	.471 (41)	.301 (28)	.228 (20)
Previous Tenure	Rent	.030 (2)	.778 (45)	.191 (12)
	Other	.194 (4)	.425 (10)	.381 (8)

Age (80+)

Note: Numbers in parentheses are unweighted cell counts. They do not yield the percentages due to weighting.

proportions are the same across age groups is rejected at the 1% level ($\chi^2 = 44.8$, 10 degrees of freedom).

Crosstabulations

In this section we concentrate on elderly homeowners and their housing transitions. The transitions fall into six categories representing housing decisions that an elderly homeowner may make:

1. move to a home with greater home equity;
2. stay in the current home with no change in status;
3. move to a home with less home equity;
4. move to a rental unit;
5. acquire a new mortgage; and
6. move into a dependent living arrangement.

This section will report results involving crosstabulations on these groups with regards to a number of financial and demographic characteristics.

Transition Definitions. The easiest housing transition to define is actually not a transition at all: Staying in one's current home with no change in tenure or mortgage status. If a homeowner reports no change in tenure status, does not move, and is not found to have acquired a mortgage, they are classified in the "Stay" category.

For those homeowners that do move and remain in the same tenure, there are separate categories for those that increase home equity (Incr) and those that decrease home equity (Decr). Home equity is calculated as the difference between reported home value and remaining mortgage principal. Unfortunately, mortgage information is unavailable in some years, and we must limit our analyses to the periods '69-'72, '76-'81, and '83-'87.

Those homeowners who move into a rental unit are placed in a fourth category (Rent). Also included in this category are the small number of homeowners who do not move but report a change in tenure status to renting, and those who report changing to a living arrangement in which housing is part of their compensation.

We are also able to distinguish a category for those homeowners who acquire a new mortgage (Mort). We identify this group as those homeowners who do not move and report that they do not have a mortgage in the former year and do have one in the latter. Also included in this category are those reporting the acquisition of a second mortgage in years in which this information is available ('69-'72, '79-'81, and '83-'87). To capture new second mortgages in the years in which they are not directly observable, and to capture those households who pay off a mortgage and acquire a new one in the same year, we include in this category households that increase their remaining mortgage principal by $20,000 or more (1987 dollars). In some cases a mortgage may be acquired exclusively for the purposes of home improvement. In these cases the new mortgage may actually *increase* home equity by increasing the home's value by more than the amount of the mortgage. Since this category seeks to identify actions that reduce home equity, we treat these cases differently: Only households who are determined to have acquired a new mortgage *and* whose home equity declines are included in the "Mort" category. Those who acquire a new mortgage and increase home equity are included in the "Stay" category.

The final category defined in these analyses is a change to a dependent living arrangement, (Dep). Most of this category is composed of those who list "other" as their tenure status and report that their housing is paid for by others in the second of the adjacent years. We also include in this category the "dependent sharers" described above, and those determined to have moved into a nursing home. Also included are a small number of households who neither own nor rent and list "temporary" or "other" as why they don't own or rent.

Transition Percentages. The weighted owner transition percentages for the total pooled sample are presented in Table 4. As one would expect, remaining in the same housing situation is by far the most common alternative chosen. Moving into a rental unit is the next most common. Among those that move to other owner-occupied housing, decreasing one's home equity is slightly more common. Reducing home equity by acquiring a new mortgage is about as likely as becoming a renter or moving to a home with less home equity. Moving into a dependent living arrangement is the alternative chosen the least. The results of Table 4 provide some evidence that homeowners may wish to dissave out of their accumulated

TABLE 4. Weighted Owner Transition Percentages

Incr	Stay	Decr	Rent	Mort	Dep
1.3%	93.5%	1.5%	1.6%	1.4%	.8%
(95)	(7631)	(122)	(128)	(143)	(69)

Note: Numbers in parentheses are unweighted cell counts. They do not yield the percentages due to weighting.

home equity. Over 5% of the pooled sample take some sort of action in adjacent years that reduces home equity.

Crosstabulation by Age Group. As an introduction to the crosstabulations, we present an age group crosstabulation in Table 5. It appears as though movements into rental situations generally increase as age increases, while acquisitions of new mortgages follow an opposite pattern. Movements into dependent relationships appear to occur in more advanced years, while no strong pattern appears in the increase or decrease categories. A chi-square test (25 degrees of freedom) rejects the null hypothesis that the transition rates do not vary across age groups ($\chi^2 = 90.1$).

Home Equity Crosstabulation. We now examine crosstabulations that capture the financial factors affecting the elderly homeowner. Table 6 presents weighted owner transition percentages by various brackets of home equity held in the year before the transition. Those in the lowest equity brackets appear to have the highest propensity of increasing their home equity by moving. They also have the highest probability of entering a dependent arrangement. There appears to be little relationship between home equity and the propensity to move to a rental unit or acquire a new mortgage. Only the propensity to move to a home of lesser equity seems to increase with home equity, and the relationship is not strong. These observations provide little support for the idea that housing changes that reduce home equity occur more often with high levels of equity. Nonetheless, a chi-square test rejects the hypothesis that there is no variation across home equity groups (35 degrees of freedom, 1% level, $\chi^2 = 65.1$). However, much of the variation upon which the hypothesis is rejected comes from categories that, if anything, run counter to intuition.

TABLE 5. Weighted Owner Transition Percentages Within Age Group

	Incr	Stay	Decr	Rent	Mort	Dep
Age						
50-59	1.2%	92.5%	2.0%	1.6%	2.5%	.2%
	(11)	(1069)	(26)	(20)	(36)	(3)
60-64	1.2%	92.7%	2.3%	1.1%	2.2%	.4%
	(17)	(1417)	(31)	(18)	(40)	(9)
65-69	1.4%	94.0%	1.3%	1.1%	1.6%	.6%
	(25)	(1772)	(23)	(21)	(35)	(12)
70-74	1.3%	95.0%	1.0%	1.4%	.7%	.6%
	(19)	(1549)	(17)	(24)	(18)	(10)
75-79	.7%	93.3%	1.2%	2.4%	.7%	1.8%
	(9)	(1012)	(12)	(26)	(9)	(20)
80+	1.7%	92.1%	1.7%	2.2%	.7%	1.6%
	(14)	(812)	(13)	(19)	(5)	(15)

Note: Numbers in parentheses are unweighted cell counts. They do not yield the percentages due to weighting.

Imputed Asset Crosstabulation. Another financial factor of interest is the effect of financial assets on homeowners' propensities to make various housing changes. As mentioned above, the PSID lacks asset data in almost all of its waves. It does record income from assets, and we use this variable to impute asset amounts for each household in each wave. The imputation is as follows: To avoid simultaneity bias, we use asset income from the initial of the two adjacent years. We assume that households hold $200 in non-interest bearing accounts. We also assume that the first $100 of interest income comes from assets earning 5% interest. Any amount above $100 is assumed to accrue from assets earning 10% interest. This procedure is admittedly crude, and later work may employ more sophisticated imputation methods.

Table 7 presents the transition percentages associated with each bracket of imputed assets. Few clear patterns are evident from an examination of Table 7. Those homeowners with high levels of assets seem generally more likely to increase their home equity.

TABLE 6. Weighted Owner Transition Percentages Within Home Equity Bracket

	Incr	Stay	Decr	Rent	Mort	Dep
Home Equity (000's 87$)						
Less Than 10	1.9% (12)	90.1% (694)	1.1% (8)	2.4% (19)	1.9% (13)	2.6% (19)
10 to 20	2.1% (18)	93.2% (936)	.8% (12)	1.1% (14)	1.3% (19)	1.4% (11)
20 to 30	1.1% (11)	93.4% (1073)	1.3% (15)	2.1% (20)	1.3% (23)	.8% (6)
30 to 40	1.3% (13)	93.9% (1019)	1.7% (18)	1.2% (15)	1.4% (18)	.6% (8)
40 to 50	.9% (7)	93.9% (857)	1.9% (17)	1.9% (18)	1.2% (19)	.2% (2)
50 to 75	1.2% (19)	93.9% (1564)	1.2% (19)	1.4% (22)	1.4% (26)	1.0% (17)
75 to 100	1.3% (10)	94.1% (779)	1.6% (13)	1.2% (10)	1.1% (13)	.6% (5)
More Than 100	.7% (5)	93.5% (709)	2.8% (20)	1.5% (10)	1.4% (12)	.1% (1)

Note: Numbers in parentheses are unweighted cell counts. They do not yield the percentages due to weighting.

A clear relationship is not evident among those that decrease equity, but moving to a rental unit or dependent arrangement seems to be somewhat inhibited by a high level of assets. The relationship between asset levels and mortgage acquisition is too weak to draw any conclusions. Despite these weak results, a chi-square test with 25 degrees of freedom rejects the hypothesis that there is no variation in housing changes among the asset groups ($\chi^2 = 76.8$).

Income Crosstabulation. As an initial analysis of this aspect, we aggregate total taxable and transfer income of the head and wife into a single summary measure of income. Table 8 presents crosstabula-

TABLE 7. Weighted Owner Transition Percentages Within Imputed Financial Asset Bracket

	Incr	Stay	Decr	Rent	Mort	Dep
Assets (000's 87$)						
Less Than 1	.8% (24)	92.5% (3094)	1.4% (47)	2.0% (62)	2.0% (88)	1.4% (43)
1 to 10	1.0% (14)	94.2% (1251)	1.5% (19)	1.6% (22)	.7% (11)	.9% (10)
10 to 30	1.0% (11)	93.7% (1030)	1.6% (17)	1.9% (19)	1.0% (13)	.7% (7)
30 to 50	1.6% (10)	93.7% (609)	1.7% (10)	.9% (8)	1.3% (9)	.7% (5)
50 to 100	2.6% (22)	93.4% (763)	1.7% (15)	1.2% (10)	1.1% (9)	0% (0)
More Than 100	1.6% (14)	94.3% (850)	1.5% (14)	.8% (7)	1.3% (11)	.5% (4)

Note: Numbers in parentheses are unweighted cell counts. They do not yield the percentages due to weighting.

tions across income groups. By examining Table 8 it appears as though income has a stimulative effect on homeowners' propensity to increase their equity by moving. No distinct pattern occurs within the decrease and new mortgage columns, but greater amounts of income appear to have an inhibiting effect on moving into a rental unit and living dependently. A chi-square test strongly rejects the hypothesis that there is no difference in change of housing status across income groups ($\chi^2 = 108.5$, 30 degrees of freedom, 1% level).

Housing Cost Crosstabulation. The final financial variable that we explore is a measure of housing costs. We construct this measure, by adding the homeowner's mortgage payment, utility payment, and property tax. In one of the relevant years utility figures are not recorded and in another property tax is not recorded. This reduces the usable sample size by about 20%. All figures are annual and come from the first of the adjacent years. Table 9 presents the

TABLE 8. Weighted Owner Transition Percentages Within Total Income Bracket

	Incr	Stay	Decr	Rent	Mort	Dep
Income (000's 87$)						
Less Than 5	.6% (4)	91.8% (875)	.6% (7)	3.0% (27)	1.8% (19)	2.3% (22)
5 to 10	1.1% (18)	92.9% (1719)	1.4% (22)	1.9% (33)	1.2% (37)	1.5% (28)
10 to 15	1.1% (13)	93.2% (1338)	1.9% (27)	1.8% (23)	1.2% (25)	.9% (10)
15 to 20	1.0% (10)	95.2% (950)	1.2% (12)	1.0% (12)	1.1% (14)	.6% (4)
20 to 30	1.1% (15)	94.4% (1220)	2.0% (26)	1.1% (14)	1.3% (18)	.2% (2)
30 to 50	1.9% (19)	94.2% (984)	1.3% (13)	1.2% (12)	1.5% (17)	0% (0)
More Than 50	2.4% (16)	91.7% (545)	2.4% (15)	1.1% (7)	1.8% (13)	.5% (3)

Note: Numbers in parentheses are unweighted cell counts. They do not yield the percentages due to weighting.

crosstabulation results. For most of the housing alternatives, the transition rates are highest at both ends of the housing cost spectrum. The only alternative that appears to follow intuition is the rental alternative, with this choice generally becoming more likely as housing costs increase. Nonetheless, and largely because of the values in the high and low brackets, a chi-square test (20 degrees of freedom, 1% level) rejects the hypothesis that the choice of housing alternative does not vary across the brackets ($\chi^2 = 66.1$).

Employment Status Crosstabulation. We now turn to several nonfinancial characteristics, the first being change in employment status. In Table 10 we classify households into four groups that describe the head of household's work status before and after the potential housing change. A number of interesting observations are

TABLE 9. Weighted Owner Transition Percentages Within Housing Cost Bracket

	Incr	Stay	Decr	Rent	Mort	Dep
Cost (000's 87$)						
Less Than 1	1.7% (14)	91.3% (813)	2.0% (15)	.9% (10)	1.7% (22)	2.3% (21)
1 to 2	1.0% (23)	94.0% (2269)	1.5% (40)	1.4% (33)	1.5% (47)	.6% (17)
2 to 3	.6% (7)	94.5% (1294)	1.3% (16)	1.8% (24)	1.3% (20)	.5% (7)
3 to 5	.7% (8)	93.9% (1051)	2.0% (22)	1.9% (22)	1.0% (14)	.5% (5)
More Than 5	2.7% (18)	91.0% (724)	2.2% (17)	1.4% (10)	2.3% (22)	.4% (4)

Note: Numbers in parentheses are unweighted cell counts. They do not yield the percentages due to weighting.

TABLE 10. Weighted Owner Transition Percentages Within Changes in Employment Status

	Incr	Stay	Decr	Rent	Mort	Dep
Employment Change						
Remains Working	1.0% (22)	94.5% (1985)	1.3% (29)	.9% (21)	2.4% (58)	.0% (1)
Becomes Working	2.6% (5)	89.9% (192)	3.0% (6)	2.1% (4)	1.5% (3)	.9% (2)
Becomes Non-Working	1.8% (7)	90.7% (431)	2.1% (9)	2.6% (11)	1.6% (9)	1.3% (5)
Remains Non-Working	1.3% (61)	93.5% (5012)	1.5% (77)	1.7% (91)	1.0% (71)	1.1% (60)

Note: Numbers in parentheses are unweighted cell counts. They do not yield the percentages due to weighting.

evident in Table 10. Households who stay employed are the least likely to make any housing change, with the exception of the acquisition of a mortgage, which they are the most likely to do. Exiting the labor force seems to be associated with moves that reduce home equity. Getting a new job is most strongly associated with movements into other owner-occupied homes, although an increase or decrease in home equity appears to be equally likely under these circumstances.

The relatively small number of households experiencing changes in employment status makes it unwise to perform a chi-square test on the data as it is. It is necessary to combine the "becomes working" and "becomes non-working" categories to achieve sufficient numbers. When this is done, the chi-square test strongly rejects the hypothesis that there is no variation across employment categories at the 1% level ($\chi^2 = 61.1$, 10 degrees of freedom).

Disability Status Crosstabulation. Another demographic characteristic that may play a large role in the elderly's housing decision is that of disability. We create a table along the lines of the previous subsection, and present the results in Table 11. Homeowners that

TABLE 11. Weighted Owner Transition Percentages Within Changes in Disability Status

	Incr	Stay	Decr	Rent	Mort	Dep
Disability Change						
Remains Well	1.3% (47)	94.5% (3482)	1.4% (58)	1.2% (45)	1.3% (64)	.3% (9)
Becomes Well	1.7% (11)	92.1% (702)	2.5% (16)	1.5% (11)	1.5% (15)	.7% (5)
Remains Limited	1.2% (27)	92.0% (2461)	1.4% (33)	2.3% (59)	1.4% (49)	1.7% (44)
Becomes Limited	1.2% (9)	94.2% (877)	1.5% (14)	.8% (10)	1.3% (15)	1.1% (11)

Note: Numbers in parentheses are unweighted cell counts. They do not yield the percentages due to weighting.

remain or become healthy are more likely to increase home equity than their limited counterparts. Becoming well also appears to stimulate movement into owner-occupied homes of lesser equity. Remaining disabled is associated with moves into rental units, but becoming disabled seems to inhibit the act of becoming a renter. No strong relationship between disability and mortgage acquisition is evident, but those remaining or becoming disabled are the most likely to enter a dependent living arrangement. A chi-square test rejects the hypothesis that there is no variation among the four disability transitions ($\chi^2 = 55.0$, 15 degrees of freedom, 1% level).

Marital Status Crosstabulation. We now turn to marital status. We classify households as married or unmarried (widowed, divorced, single) in the years before and after a potential move, resulting in a total of four categories. The results are presented in Table 12. Remaining married seems to have a stabilizing effect on a household's housing arrangements, and particularly seems to inhibit moves into rental units and dependency. Becoming married is associated with moves into other owner-occupied arrangements, although the numbers are too small in this category to lead us to strong conclusions. Remaining unmarried seems to encourage moves into rental units and dependency. Becoming unmarried is

TABLE 12. Weighted Owner Transition Percentages Within Changes in Marital Status

	Incr	Stay	Decr	Rent	Mort	Dep
Marital Change						
Remains Married	1.5% (63)	94.4% (4262)	1.6% (72)	.8% (36)	1.4% (82)	.3% (12)
Becomes Married	5.2% (1)	76.5% (18)	18.2% (4)	0% (0)	.2% (1)	0% (0)
Remains Unmarried	.9% (28)	92.9% (3169)	1.1% (37)	2.4% (82)	1.3% (54)	1.4% (50)
Becomes Unmarried	1.5% (3)	83.3% (182)	5.1% (9)	4.3% (10)	2.2% (6)	3.5% (7)

Note: Numbers in parentheses are unweighted cell counts. They do not yield the percentages due to weighting.

strongly associated with all types of housing changes, but especially ones that reduce home equity. Again the numbers in some categories are very small. In this case, combining the categories would not be meaningful because the categories describe very different things, and thus we do not perform the chi-square test.

Children Crosstabulation. The final demographic characteristic deals with the effect of children on a homeowner's housing decision. We define this characteristic as a change in the number of children living in the household in the adjacent years (see Table 13). Those households that experience no change in the number of children are divided into those that have children (present), and those that don't (not present).

Those that have children and experience no change in the number of children tend to be less likely to increase home equity, and more likely to acquire a new mortgage. In those households where the number of children decreases, moves to homes having less equity, rental units, and the acquisition of a new mortgage are more common. This suggests a somewhat strong "empty nest" effect is pres-

TABLE 13. Weighted Owner Transition Percentages Within Changes in Number of Children

	Incr	Stay	Decr	Rent	Mort	Dep
Number of Children						
No Change	1.3%	93.6%	1.5%	1.6%	1.2%	.8%
(not present)	(88)	(6547)	(100)	(110)	(94)	(61)
No Change	.6%	94.0%	1.3%	1.0%	2.7%	.4%
(present)	(5)	(712)	(12)	(8)	(24)	(2)
Decrease	.2%	90.7%	2.9%	2.5%	3.0%	.8%
	(1)	(290)	(7)	(10)	(17)	(3)
Increase	1.5%	84.0%	3.9%	0%	6.5%	4.1%
	(1)	(82)	(3)	(0)	(8)	(3)

Note: Numbers in parentheses are unweighted cell counts. They do not yield the percentages due to weighting.

ent. Those households that experience an increase in the number of children tend to move to lower equity homes and acquire new mortgages more often. Although these results are suggestive, the small numbers in some categories make a rigorous statistical test impossible.

DISCUSSION

Discussion of Results

The simple results of this paper suggest that demographic considerations may be more important than financial considerations to elderly homeowners' housing decisions. Crosstabulations on marital, employment, children, and disability factors yield strong, intuitively consistent results as to their effect on housing changes. Financial variables, on the other hand, have less consistent results. Home equity and housing costs do not have consistently strong relationships across housing transitions. Where they do have relationships, they are often different from what is indicated by intuition. The results for income and financial assets are somewhat better, but are not particularly strong. Overall these results suggest that demographic factors are much more important than financial factors in elderly homeowners' housing decisions.

Critique of the Results

Consistent Statistical Significance of Results. The reader should not interpret the unanimous rejection of null hypotheses as evidence that all of these factors are important determinants of the elderly's housing behavior. The null hypotheses put forth are that there is no relationship between a particular variable and housing changes. Thus even relationships that run counter to those expected contribute to the rejection of the null. One should also be aware that the sample size examined is large. This causes statistical significance to occur more frequently than with samples of smaller size. Therefore we may find a very weak and behaviorally insignificant relationship to be statistically significant. A final reason for viewing the test statistics suspiciously is that the data come from pooled cross sections. Since a single household may contribute multiple observations, the sample could be viewed as not being independent. If households behave similarly year to year they may reduce the variation observed in the sample and increase the size of the test statistic.

Correlation Among Factors. Many of the variables examined here are likely to be correlated with one another. This is especially true among the variables that perform the worst, the financial ones. The correlation, if present, may obscure underlying relationships in some cases and lead to misleading results in others. For example, home equity and financial assets may be highly correlated and the single dimension crosstabulations may confuse relationships that would be evident in a multidimensional analysis. Home equity is also likely to be correlated with the size of the home and the length of tenure in the home, both of which may work counter to the effects of home equity. Rather than attempting to control for correlation within the context of crosstabulations, we will employ multivariate regressions in later work.

Other Determinants. A number of potentially important factors are not examined in this article. Specifically, housing characteristics may play a significant role. Although there is not a strong consensus, several authors (Lane and Feins, 1985; Béland, 1984; Lawton, 1980; O'Bryant and Wolf, 1983) have found interesting results regarding the effects of number of rooms, years lived in the home, and some measures of housing quality. There is also some work examining the psychological value of home ownership (O'Bryant, 1982; Lawton, 1980; Reschovsky, 1990). The data used in this analysis are taken over a long time period in which interest rates, inflation, and home equity appreciation varied greatly. A more complete analysis would attempt to include these considerations.

FUTURE WORK

The results of this article suggest that a number of factors have significant effects on a number of very different housing changes. They also suggest that financial factors pale in comparison to the effect of demographic factors when it comes to the elderly's home ownership decisions. While the results are suggestive, they still do not provide completely convincing evidence that demographic factors are dominant, or that financial factors are irrelevant. To gain better insight on these questions we will employ multivariate regression analyses. These analyses will include a number of factors not seen here, such as housing characteristics (number of rooms, type of dwelling unit, length of tenure) and additional demographic characteristics (gender, education, support from relatives). These improvements should add to our understanding of the housing decisions of elderly homeowners.

REFERENCES

Ai, C., Feinstein, J., McFadden, D., & Pollakowski, H. (1990). The Dynamics of Housing Demand by the Elderly: User Cost Effects. In D. Wise (ed.), *Issues in the Economics of Aging*. Chicago: University of Chicago Press.

American Housing Survey 1985: National Core File Documentation. (1987). Washington, DC: U.S. Department of Commerce, Bureau of the Census.

American Housing Survey for the United States in 1987. (1989). Washington, DC: U.S. Department of Commerce, Bureau of the Census.

Béland, F. (1984). The Decision of Elderly Persons to Leave Their Homes. *The Gerontologist, 24*, pp. 179-185.

Boersch-Supan, A. (1989). A Dynamic Analysis of Household Dissolution and Living Arrangement Transitions by Elderly Americans. *NBER Working Paper* #2808. Cambridge, MA: National Bureau of Economic Research.

Boersch-Supan, A., Hajivassiliou, V., Kotlikoff, L.J., & Morris, J.M. (1990). Health, Children, and Elderly Living Arrangements: A Multiperiod-Multinomial Probit Model with Unobserved Heterogeneity and Autocorrelated Errors. *NBER Working Paper* #3343. Cambridge, MA: National Bureau of Economic Research.

Boersch-Supan, A., Kotlikoff, L.J., and Morris, J.N. (1988). The Dynamics of Living Arrangements of the Elderly. *NBER Working Paper* #2787. Cambridge, MA: National Bureau of Economic Research.

Danziger, S., Schwartz, S., & Smolensky, E. (1984). The Choice of Living Arrangements by the Elderly. In H. Aaron and G. Burtless (eds.), *Retirement and Economic Behavior*. Washington, DC: Brookings Institution.

Ellwood, D., & Kane, T. (1989). The American Way of Aging: An Event History Analysis. *NBER Working Paper* #2892. Cambridge, MA: National Bureau of Economic Research.

Feinstein, J., & McFadden, D. (1987). The Dynamics of Housing Demand by the Elderly: Wealth, Cash Flow, and Demographic Effects. *NBER Working Paper* #2471. Cambridge, MA: National Bureau of Economic Research.

Garber, A.M., and MaCurdy, T. (1989). Nursing Home Utilization Among the High-Risk Elderly. *Hoover Institution Working Paper* E-89-1. Stanford, CA: Hoover Institution, Stanford University.

Jacobs, B. (1986). The National Potential of Home Equity Conversion. *The Gerontologist, 26,* pp. 496-504.

Kotlikoff, L.J., & Morris, J. (1988). Why Don't the Elderly Live with Their Children? A New Look. *NBER Working Paper #2734.* Cambridge, MA: National Bureau of Economic Research.

Lane, T.S., & Feins, J.D. (1985). Are the Elderly Overhoused? Definitions of Space Utilization and Policy Implications. *The Gerontologist, 25,* pp. 243-250.

Lawton, M.P. (1980). Housing the Elderly. *Research on Aging, 2,* pp. 309-327.

Manchester, J. (1987). Reverse Mortgages and Their Effects on Consumption. *Dartmouth College Working Paper #87-3.* Hanover, NH: Dartmouth College.

Merrill, S. (1984). Home Equity and the Elderly. In H. Aaron and G. Burtless (eds.), *Retirement and Economic Behavior.* Washington, DC: Brookings Institution.

O'Bryant, S.L. (1982). The Value on Home to Older Persons. *Research on Aging, 4,* pp. 349-363.

O'Bryant, S.L., & Wolf, S.M. (1983). Explanations of Housing Satisfaction of Older Homeowners and Renters. *Research on Aging, 5,* pp. 217-233.

Panel Study of Income Dynamics: Procedures and Tape Codes 1987 Interviewing Year. (1989). Ann Arbor, MI: Institute for Social Research, University of Michigan.

Panel Study of Income Dynamics User's Guide. (1973). Ann Arbor, MI: Institute for Social Research, University of Michigan.

Providential Home Income Plan (PHIP). (1989). Lifetime Reverse Mortgage Consumer Information for Seniors. (Informational Flier). San Francisco, CA.

Reschovsky, J.D. (1990). Residential Immobility of the Elderly: An Empirical Investigation. *AREUEA Journal, 18,* pp. 160-183.

Retirement History Longitudinal Survey Documentation. (1986). Washington, DC: U.S. Social Security Administration.

Scholen, K., & Chen, Y. (1980). *Unlocking Home Equity for the Elderly.* New York: Ballinger Publishing.

Stahl, K. (1989). Housing Patterns and Mobility of the Aged: The United States and West Germany. In D. Wise (ed.), *The Economics of Aging.* Chicago: University of Chicago Press.

Stoller, E.P., & Stoller, M.A. (1987). The Propensity to Save Among the Elderly. *The Gerontologist, 27,* pp. 314-320.

Venti, S., & Wise, D. (1989). Aging, Moving, and Housing Wealth. In D. Wise (ed.), *The Economics of Aging.* Chicago: University of Chicago Press.

Venti, S., & Wise, D. (1990). But They Don't Want to Reduce Housing Equity. In D. Wise (ed.), *Issues in the Economics of Aging.* Chicago: University of Chicago Press.

Weinrobe, M.D. (1984). Home Equity Conversion: Its Practice Today. In *Long-Term Care Financing and Delivery Systems: Exploring Alternatives,* (Conference Proceedings). Washington, DC: U.S. Department of Health and Human Services.

Chapter 3

Elderly Housing Assistance Programs: How They Affect the Own versus Rent Decisions

Krisandra A. Guidry
James D. Shilling

SUMMARY. Elderly homeowners–age 65 and older–eventually must decide whether to own or rent. Renting may be appropriate for someone who has an alternative need or use for the money that would otherwise be tied up as equity in a home. Owning, on the other hand, often ties down the shelter costs for elderly households and provides them with greater choices to better satisfy their space needs.

I. INTRODUCTION

For many young families, the decision to own or rent a dwelling eventually becomes an important question. However, many elderly

Krisandra A. Guidry is affiliated with the Department of Economics and Finance, Nicholls State University, Thibodaux, LA 70301. James D. Shilling is affiliated with the Department of Real Estate and Urban Land Economics, University of Wisconsin-Madison, Madison, WI 53706.

[Haworth co-indexing entry note]: "Elderly Housing Assistance Programs: How They Affect the Own versus Rent Decisions." Guidry, Krisandra A., and James D. Shilling. Co-published simultaneously in *Journal of Housing for the Elderly* (The Haworth Press, Inc.) Vol. 11, No. 2, 1995, pp. 37-49; and: *Housing Decisions for the Elderly: To Move or Not to Move* (ed: Leon A. Pastalan), The Haworth Press, Inc., 1995, pp. 37-49. Multiple copies of this article/chapter may be purchased from The Haworth Document Delivery Center [1-800-3-HAWORTH; 9:00 a.m. - 5:00 p.m. (EST)].

households–age 65 and older–confront similar decisions. Elderly households who continue to own often do so because owning ties down their shelter costs. Home ownership provides elderly households with greater choices to better satisfy their space needs. To illustrate, many elderly households have special needs, such as accessibility to health care services, sites with ramps, grab bars, and the removal of interior thresholds to accommodate wheelchairs and walkers, as well as specific preferences for living near family and friends, that are best met by owning. By the same token, someone needing money for medical expenses, for example, is probably justified in selling his or her existing home and in renting a place to live.

In deciding to own or not to own, elderly households should consider direct housing assistance programs sponsored by the government. A strong case can be made for renting based on direct housing assistance programs designed specifically for elderly households.

Therefore, in this paper, we undertake the following plan of investigation. The second section looks at the major housing subsidy programs available to senior citizens. The next section examines why the elderly are different. The decision model whether to participate in assistance programs is contained in the fourth section. The fifth section presents simulation analysis. A conclusion follows.

II. THE MAJOR SUBSIDY PROGRAMS

The increasing number of older persons in the nation's population is one force behind an expanding demand for housing. Table 1 shows past and projected trends in the number of elderly citizens. It is estimated that the number of Americans 65 years of age and older will increase from 30 to 39 million between 1989 and 2010. Over the same time period, citizens aged 75 and over will increase by 50%–constituting over 6% of the entire population.

Programs subsidizing the elderly for housing were specifically outlined in the Housing Act of 1959. Its scope was further expanded by the Older Americans Act of 1965 and other bits of legislation passed by Congress granting authorization to the Department of Housing and Urban Development (HUD).

HUD has been primarily responsible for the construction of ade-

TABLE 1. Projections of the Elderly Population: 1989 to 2010

(000)

	65–74 years	75 years & older
1989	18,129	12,863
1990	18,373	13,187
1995	18,930	14,834
2000	18,243	16,639
2005	18,410	17,864
2010	21,039	18,323

Source: U.S. Bureau of the Census, *Current Population Reports*, series P–25, No. 1018.

quate housing through direct loans and loan guarantees. The major HUD programs include: low rent public housing, Section 8 (low and moderate income housing), Section 202 (rental housing assistance payments), and Section 236 (multifamily rental housing).

Other subsidy programs include the rural housing program of the Farmer's Home Administration (FmHA) and housing vouchers. This section takes a closer look at these programs.

Low Rent Public Housing

Low rent public housing, or "project" housing as it is commonly called, is owned and operated by a local housing authority. They can build new housing structures, rehabilitate old ones, buy units from builders, or lease units from individual owners.

The units are leased to families based on economic need. Tenant rent is less than market rent because the federal government not only incurs development costs during construction or rehabilitation, but also pays part of the operating expenses. This federal subsidy is comprised of annual contributions made to cover the debt service on the bonds of the local housing authority.

Section 8 Housing

The Section 8 program, authorized by the Housing and Community Development Act of 1974, consists of two distinct parts. One part has to do with existing housing, whether or not in need of moderate or substantial rehabilitation. In this program, an eligible household could actually choose its present dwelling as a subsidized unit. After inspection of the property and agreement of the landlord to participate in the program, a market rent is negotiated. The tenant then consents to pay a certain percentage of his income (30%) toward the rent; the public housing agency that administers the program pays the balance. The second part of Section 8, the new construction program, has the same payment formula; however, HUD chooses the dwellings that participate in the subsidies.

Section 202 Housing

The Section 202 assistance program is structured so as to subsidize new construction for the elderly and handicapped. The program provides loans to developers at a rate below the U.S. Treasury's long term borrowing rate and a Section 8 subsidy for each 202 unit. The program also offers direct loans for the elderly and handicapped in need of adequate housing.

Section 236 Housing

Section 236 provides subsidies to reduce the interest paid by mortgagors for multi-family housing projects, which in turn, reduces rents to tenants.

FmHA Rural Housing Program

Besides HUD, the Farmers Home Administration (FmHA) has also shown a concern in providing adequate housing for the elderly and for those with low and moderate incomes. Assistance consists primarily of loans to qualified applicants interested in building, purchasing, or repairing apartment-type housing in the open country and rural communities of up to 20,000 inhabitants.

Additional financial aid in the form of home ownership loans, building site loans, self-help housing loans, and repair loans are also available from FmHA for low and moderate income families.

Housing Vouchers

Originally developed in the 1930's, the concept of housing vouchers did not gain nationwide attention until the Reagan administration sought to cut spending on social programs. Housing vouchers are actually allowances made to low income families to help meet their monthly rents. Under a housing voucher program, local housing authorities have the ability to grant vouchers to eligible families. Tenants then agree to pay a certain percentage of their incomes toward rent; the housing authority pays the difference between a family's fixed percentage and the market rent for homes of the same size and quality.

III. WHY THE ELDERLY ARE DIFFERENT

The need for adequate housing is a necessity shared by young and old alike. Such housing should provide shelter, be accessible at a reasonable price, and cater to the "special" requirements of its occupants. Special requirements for the elderly include health status, household size and composition, and income level and asset holdings.

Among the more important of these special requirements, particularly for the elderly, is health. Being elderly is not synonymous with death and disease. However, aging does bring about a certain decline in functioning and an increase in the risk of chronic disease. It has been estimated that only 14% of the nation's elderly are free of any serious illness (Zais, Struyk and Thibodeau, 1982). Therefore, health problems by the elderly suggest that they place special demands on the environment in which they live, such as ramps, grab bars, and the removal of interior thresholds to accommodate wheelchairs and walkers.

Another special requirement of the elderly has to do with their living arrangements acting as a social environment. There is fairly strong evidence that individuals sort themselves into living arrangements depending on how much social support is needed from their environments.

The elderly who live alone, either out of choice or necessity, are often "environmentally impoverished." Housing defects, relatively common among this group, are associated with high rates of rental occupancy and constrained budgets. The housing for older women living alone is often better than housing for older men living alone, even though the poverty rates are higher for older women single person households (Zais, Struyk and Thibodeau, 1982).

Compared with the elderly who live alone, those who share living quarters with others may be poorer individually, but are less likely to live in inadequate housing or poverty. They have been found to live in newer units with fewer structural defects (Zais, Struyk and Thibodeau, 1982). Therefore, it seems clear that elderly who live with others give up independence and autonomy for better physical surroundings and richer social environments.

Income is another piece in the puzzle of problems faced by the elderly. Table 2 has figures on the money income of households–those under 65 years and those 65 years and over. Income typically falls significantly at retirement.

However, the vast majority of older people–about 70%–own their own homes (Salins, 1987). Older married couples are more likely to own homes of substantial value with paid up mortgages than unmarried elders are. Based on the value of the home and its equity, this group has a strong asset position, even though their current incomes may be weak. This can be seen in Table 3, which presents household net worth by age of householder.

TABLE 2. Money Income of Households: 1980 to 1987

- -

	Age of Householder:	
	Under 65 years	65 years old & older
After-Tax Household Income		
1980	$24,327	$15,145
1983	24,628	16,752
1984	25,278	17,228
1985	25,738	17,113
1986	26,467	17,425
1987	26,915	17,284

- -

Source: U.S. Bureau of the Census, *Current Population Reports*, series P–23, No. 157.

TABLE 3. Household Net Worth: 1988

percent distribution of households by net worth	Age of Householder (in years)				
	< 35	35-44	45-54	55-64	> 65
zero or negative	19.4	11.3	8.2	6.4	5.2
$1 to $4,999	27.6	13.3	10.5	7.5	8.9
$5,000 to $9,999	11.4	6.4	4.5	2.5	3.1
$10,000 to $24,999	16.2	13.4	9.1	7.4	8.1
$25,000 to $49,999	11.1	15.3	13.7	12.6	13.2
$50,000 to $99,999	8.0	18.2	21.1	20.5	20.9
$100,000 to $249,999	4.8	15.8	21.9	27.5	26.1
$250,000 or over	1.5	6.5	11.1	15.6	14.4

Source: U.S. Bureau of the Census, *Current Population Reports*, series P–70, No. 22.

IV. WHETHER TO PARTICIPATE IN DIRECT ASSISTANCE PROGRAMS

Obviously, not all the elderly can take advantage of governmental assistance, but for those that are eligible, the result is that it is almost always wiser to do so. For older Americans, the decision whether or not to participate in these federal assistance programs boils down to a net present value (NPV) problem. The net present value of an investment is the present value of the future benefits minus the cost. In other words, it is the difference between what is to be received, in current or present value, and what will be paid for it.

Consider the following two scenarios: elderly households who already rent and elderly households who own. For those elderly households who are already renting, the switch to subsidized housing is often the optimal thing to do. Participation in, say, the Section 8 program or a similar program can produce cost savings of 5-10 percent, on average, for the typical elderly household (Salins, 1987).

For those elderly households who currently are homeowners, the problem is more complicated. On the one hand, most elderly home-owners have no mortgage debt outstanding at this point in their lives, so that the direct out-of-pocket costs and expenses of home ownership are fairly minimal. On the other hand, while the elderly must live somewhere, home ownership does not necessarily follow. Renting a dwelling unit is certainly appropriate for many elderly households who have an alternative need or use for the money that would otherwise be tied up as equity in a home. Furthermore, rent-ing may be desirable if households could lower their housing ex-penditures by participating in direct housing assistance programs designed specifically for the elderly.

When presented with the choice between owning and renting a subsidized unit, an elderly homeowner should be indifferent at a level of rent where the payment savings from participating in the direct housing assistance program plus the interest earnings on the sales proceeds of the house exactly equal any forgone housing appreciation from owning.

To illustrate, suppose Joe Olfolkes, a retired Des Moines, Iowa, machinist, and his wife Ida each turn 65 this year. Based on health exams, they are expected to be able to live on their own for the next ten years. Their combined monthly income from Social Security is $730 ($8760 a year). In their 40 years of marriage to one another, Joe and Ida have amassed a moderate asset position. Earnings per year from investments (CDs, stocks, and bonds) are negligible. However, the largest asset in their portfolio is their home. Pur-chased over 30 years ago, there is no longer any mortgage debt outstanding on the house. Now that their four children are grown and married with families of their own, the Olfolkes must ask themselves which situation proves most beneficial to their pocketbooks–continuing to own their home until moving to a nursing home or perhaps selling it, then moving to a subsidized rental unit until they are ready for a care facility.

The decision can be easily made by preparing a cost-benefit analysis. If Joe and Ida choose to sell the house and move to a rental unit for the next ten years, the cost associated with doing so, ignoring expenses and tax exemptions, is the forgone housing appreciation. We assume the following: The house and the property will have a market value at the time of the sale of $125,000. The housing appreciation rate in this area is 2%. By selling the home now, the Olfolkes forgo an increase of 2% per year in the price of their home ($125,000 × 2% = $2500 per year).

Investment of the sales proceeds should yield the current market interest rate, which is assumed to be 8%. This translates into $10,000 per year additional income ($125,000 × .08 = $10,000).

In addition, we assume that the current market rent for a suitable apartment in this area is $583 per month, or $7000 per year.

The differential cash flow benefits of the direct assistance programs involve the subtraction of the rents under the direct assistance program, 30% of the Olfolkes total yearly income (30% of social security and interest payments), $5628, from the rents in the absence of housing subsidies, $7000 per year in this case.

Both costs and benefits are then discounted at the current market interest rate over the time period in question < 10 years in this case) in order to obtain their present values. Table 4 gives an accounting of these costs and benefits for Joe and Ida's home.

The net present value of participating in assistance programs is simply the present value of the benefits minus the present value of the costs. If the net present value of participating in assistance programs is greater (less) than zero, then the homeowner is better (worse) off selling his property than keeping it. It can be seen from the tabulations that Joe and Ida should sell their home and move to a subsidized unit for the next ten years since NPV > 0.

V. SIMULATION ANALYSIS

Simulation analysis indicates exactly how much NPV will change in response to a given change in an input variable, other

TABLE 4. Costs and Benefits of Participating in Direct Assistance Program

- -

Time period (n)	10 years

Costs of Direct Assistance Program

Forgone housing appreciation ($125,000 × .02)	$ 2,500 (per year)

Benefits of Direct Assistance Program

Rents in absence of housing subsidies	$7,000
− Rents under direct assistance program	5,628
Payment savings due to assistance program	1,372
+ Interest earnings on sales proceeds	10,000
Total benefits of direct assistance program	$11,372 (per year)

Present value of costs $= $ Forgone housing appreciation $\times$ $PVAF_{i\%, n}$*

$\qquad = \$2,500 \times PVAF_{8\%, 10}$

$\qquad = \$2,500 \times 6.7101$

$\qquad = \$16,775$

Present value of benefits $=$ Total benefits of direct assistance programs $\times PVAF_{i\%, n}$*

$\qquad = \$11,372 \times PVAF_{8\%, 10}$

$\qquad = \$11,372 \times 6.7101$

$\qquad = \$76,307$

Net present value of participating in assistance program

$\qquad =$ Present value of benefits − Present value of costs

$\qquad = \$76,307 - \$16,775$

$\qquad = \$59,532$

Since NPV > 0, the property should be sold.

- -

*The present value of an annuity is the value today of a series of equal payments paid every year for n years in the future, discounted at i%. Tables have been constructed for the present value annuity factor (PVAF) for various values of i and n. See Brigham and Gapenski (1988) for a complete set of tables.

things held constant. Table 5 is the base case scenario for various housing appreciation rates and interest rates. The homeowner's yearly income from Social Security is $8760 per year, while the current market rent for an apartment is $7000 per year. It is assumed that the property (home) is sold at a price of $100,000. The occupants then move to a subsidized unit for the next seven years. The rents under the direct assistance program and the interest earnings on the sales proceeds change as the interest rates change. In certain situations, i.e., when housing appreciation rates are high and interest rates are low, the decision to participate in assistance programs has a NPV less than zero and is not the preferred alternative.

Meanwhile, Table 6, with much of the same assumptions as Table 5, shows how the decision to participate in assistance programs is affected by various holding periods. Panel A assumes that the home is sold and the occupants move to a subsidized unit for the next 4 years. In Panel B, the occupants live in a subsidized unit for 12 years. As before, the NPV of participating in assistance programs is positive for most housing appreciation rates. However, the NPV's are smaller for the shorter time period. As the time period is extended, the NPV's increase.

TABLE 5. NPV of Participating in Direct Housing Assistance Programs for Elderly Homeowners: Base Case Scenario*

Interest Rate	Housing Appreciation Rate				
	2%	4%	6%	8%	10%
6%	$36,687	$25,522	$14,358	$3,193	$(7,972)
8%	41,505	31,092	20,680	10,267	(146)
10%	45,626	35,889	26,153	16,416	6,679
12%	47,335	38,208	29,080	19,953	10,825
14%	52,197	43,621	35,044	26,468	17,891

*A positive NPV in this table indicates that elderly homeowners would be better off at this point in their lives renting a subsidized dwelling unit. For example, if the housing appreciation rate were 4% and current interest rates were 10%, an elderly household could earn an additional $35,889 over the next 7 years by moving to a subsidized dwelling unit and investing the proceeds from sale at 10% interest.

TABLE 6. Impact of Time Period on the NPV of Participating in Direct Housing Assistance Programs for Elderly Homeowners

	Panel A: 4-year Time Period Housing Appreciation Rate				
Interest Rate	2%	4%	6%	8%	10%
6%	$22,773	$15,843	$8,912	$1,982	$(4,948)
8%	26,404	19,780	13,198	6,531	(93)
10%	29,708	23,368	17,029	10,689	4,349
12%	31,502	25,428	19,353	13,279	7,204
14%	35,466	29,638	23,811	17,983	12,156

	Panel B: 12-year Time Period Housing Appreciation Rate				
Interest Rate	2%	4%	6%	8%	10%
6%	$55,098	$38,331	$21,563	$4,796	$(11,972)
8%	60,078	45,006	29,933	14,861	(211)
10%	63,858	50,230	36,603	22,975	9,348
12%	64,248	51,859	39,471	27,082	14,693
14%	68,897	57,577	46,256	34,936	23,615

*A positive NPV in this table indicates that elderly homeowners would be better off at this point in their lives renting a subsidized dwelling unit.

VI. CONCLUSION

Elderly homeowners–age 65 or older–eventually must decide whether to own or rent. Renting may be appropriate for someone who has an alternative need or use for the money that would otherwise be tied up as equity in a home. Owning, on the other hand, often ties down the shelter costs for elderly households and provides them with greater choices to satisfy better their space needs.

In deciding whether or not to own, elderly households should consider direct housing assistance programs sponsored by the government. The Department of Housing and Urban Development

(HUD) has primarily been responsible for the construction of elderly rental housing through direct loans and loan guarantees. HUD programs include: Public Housing, Section 8, Section 202, and Section 236. Besides HUD, the Farmers Home Administration (FmHA) and housing vouchers have provided adequate housing for the elderly.

For older Americans, the decision whether or not to participate in these federal assistance programs boils down to a net present value problem. They must ask themselves which situation proves most beneficial to their pocketbooks–continuing to own their home until moving to a nursing home or perhaps selling it and moving into a subsidized rental unit. The decision can be easily made by preparing a cost-benefit analysis. Simulations illustrate that the decision to participate in assistance programs is sometimes most beneficial to the elderly depending on the value of certain variables such as interest rates, housing appreciation rates, and length of the holding period.

REFERENCES

Brigham, E.F. and Gapenski, L.C. (1988). *Financial Management: Theory and Practice.* Chicago: Dryden Press.

Salins, P.D. (1987). "America's Permanent Housing Problem," in *Housing America's Poor,* P.D. Salins, ed. Chapel Hill, NC: University of North Carolina.

Zais, J.P., Struyk, R.J. and Thibodeau, T. (1982). *Housing Assistance for Older Americans.* Washington: Urban Institute.

Chapter 4

Selecting Senior Housing: Information Needs and Sources

Leslie A. Morgan
Constance Krach

SUMMARY. How do consumers and professionals go about locating appropriate housing for older adults unable to live independently, what information do they seek, what do housing providers want to know, and do consumers know the key questions to ask? This pilot study examines these issues with data gathered from a sample of housing providers and from focus groups of older adults.
Many older consumers do not have a clear idea of where to turn for information on housing. Cost and services are the most central issues to consumers, while professionals focus on functional impairment and space availability.

With the growth of the elderly population, especially those over 85, the problem of locating appropriate supportive housing environments will be faced by more older persons and their families (Rabin &

Leslie A. Morgan, PhD, is Professor of Sociology, University of Maryland Baltimore County, 5401 Wilkens Avenue, Baltimore, MD 21228-5398. Constance Krach, MA, recently completed her Master's Degree in Sociology at the University of Maryland Baltimore County.

Support for this research was provided by NIA Grant R43 AG10341. Support for computer analyses was provided by the Office of Academic Computing, University of Maryland Baltimore County.

[Haworth co-indexing entry note]: "Selecting Senior Housing: Information Needs and Sources." Morgan, Leslie A., and Constance Krach. Co-published simultaneously in *Journal of Housing for the Elderly* (The Haworth Press, Inc.) Vol. 11, No. 2, 1995, pp. 51-66; and: *Housing Decisions for the Elderly: To Move or Not to Move* (ed: Leon A. Pastalan) The Haworth Press, Inc., 1995, pp. 51-66. Multiple copies of this article/chapter may be purchased from The Haworth Document Delivery Center [1-800-3-HAWORTH; 9:00 a.m. - 5:00 p.m. (EST)].

Stockton, 1987). Needs of those seeking housing must be matched with the options available in the marketplace, a difficult process under the best of circumstances (Ehrlich, 1986). Searches are even more difficult for special needs sub-populations, who may need housing at the bottom end of the market and lack advocates and resources (Huff, 1986; Pynoos, 1987)

Often a housing search occurs in a crisis, where an impending release from a hospital or sudden illness necessitates quick relocation (Ambrogi, 1991). In other cases, such as dementia, loss of spouse, or anticipated health decline, the process of locating supportive housing may be undertaken more slowly and planfully. In both situations, however, the choice of housing is viewed as key to life satisfaction and maintenance of healthful functioning of the older person (Kahana, 1974; Lawton, 1980).

This paper provides findings from a pilot study on how consumers seek housing, what information they need, and what housing providers see occurring during this information-seeking and person/environment matching process.

CURRENT LITERATURE ON HOUSING SEARCHES

A review of the literature found surprisingly limited information pertaining directly to the process of selecting housing once a relocation decision had been made. The literature discusses the problems leading to that decision and problems of adjustment following a relocation. But little is said of how the older person, along with kin and professionals, moves from defining the need to selecting a particular housing alternative. Specifically, little is known about the resources used and the information needed in making appropriate housing selections (Mansbach, 1988).

Specialized Housing Needs of Frail Elders

Selecting supportive housing is not simply a matter of preference. Specialized environmental features (e.g., wheelchair access, security for wanderers) as well as the services to residents (e.g., meals, personal care) determine the appropriateness of a setting (Lawton, 1985). Health status, resource limitations and the supply of available housing/care settings determine the realistic options (Daily, 1987).

A Canadian study of interest in relocation showed that those wishing to leave their homes lacked resources to stay in them, had recent functional health declines, were concerned about safety, and had difficulty in functioning during winter months (Beland, 1984). Sherman's research (1971) on elders' motivation for moving into age-specialized housing suggests that limited demands for maintenance, care for health and personal needs, and diminishing physical strength were all factors in relocation from their prior residence. Other characteristics that influenced site selection were nearness to facilities and services, cost, access to kin and friends, and recreational facilities (Sherman, 1971).

Butler and associates (1983) describe the British system of sheltered housing, where needs are assessed and space in units is (theoretically) allocated on that basis. This need evaluation, however, is highly subjective and other factors, such as the demands of current clients in that setting, help to determine placement decisions. Social workers and physicians may overstate the level of client independence in order to secure a placement in sheltered housing. Further, persons deciding placement are often uninvolved with the consequences of a poor match, and thus are not invested in making certain that a good fit of person to environment is made (Butler et al., 1983).

Research has discussed difficulties, such as loss of function and excess costs, that can arise from placement in an overly-restrictive environment (see Sherwood et al., 1986). The goal of the process is fitting the older person in the least restrictive environment that meets their physical, cognitive, and social needs (Ehrlich, 1986) along the continuum from independent community living to skilled nursing facilities (Sherwood et al., 1986). The continuum of care theoretically provides a range of housing alternatives with varying levels of support. Individuals with increasing needs may move from one level to the next as the need arises, assuming that space at the next level is available and affordable, and that clients know of its existence (Bernstein, 1982). Some argue that the function of a continuum of care, to the extent it exists in particular areas, requires mechanisms for steering elderly individuals to the appropriate setting (Anderson et al., 1984).

Searching for Appropriate Alternatives

Housing is currently located in various ways. The elderly person or family members may contact providers directly or work through agency or private referral programs. Others are assisted by health care or social work professionals. State and local agencies offer listings of licensed or certified housing of various types in their areas. More disadvantaged individuals, with fewer options due to financial constraints, may be lucky to locate any supportive housing to accept them at all (Ehrlich, 1986).

The information provided in provider lists typically omits issues such as the availability of space, services provided and eligibility requirements, which can be determined only by direct contact with the housing provider. Family members, the elderly, and other professionals working with them encounter an incomplete informational system and a labor-intensive process of contacting individual service providers to determine whether there is a good client/facility match (Anderson et al., 1984).

Physicians, who often make relocation recommendations, are unlikely to be aware of the range of non-medical supportive housing options available in the community (King & Collins, 1990; U.S. Congress, 1990). Social workers, who should be key professionals in the process of housing location, have written little on the topic, except to reinforce the importance of matching elders to their environments (Helen & Griffiths, 1983; Sherman & Newman, 1979). Placement in adult foster care is typically mediated by a social worker (Sherman & Newman, 1979). Knowledge of the special traits of both caregivers and potential residents is key in this more intimate environment, but social workers often fail to fulfill their potentials in these mediating roles (Sherman & Newman, 1979). Inadequate knowledge about housing options among both informal and formal advisors to elders seeking housing could result in less adequate placements and lower subsequent functioning and satisfaction.

Determinants of Level of Care

One study attempted to quantify factors determining the level of supportive housing required by aged persons. Six dimensions predicted the need for supportive housing: confusion, physical dependency, need for meal services, anxiety, current residence in dependent living arrangement, and lack of peer group socialization (Sherwood et al., 1975). This study suggested that moderately trained individuals, asking specific questions in a screening interview, could determine the information needed to make a suitable choice. Others have developed checklists for deinstitutionalized individuals with chronic mental illness to maximize the fit between the person and their housing environment (Betts et al., 1981).

On the other side of the process, those responsible for admission and retention decisions in housing are well aware of their questions and requirements for potential residents (Barker et al., 1988; Bernstein, 1982; Heumann, 1988; Sherman & Newman, 1979). A growing body of literature discusses decisions of housing managers to relocate increasingly frail tenants, but much less regarding how that process actually takes place (Barker et al., 1988; Bernstein, 1982; Heumann, 1988). There remain many unknowns regarding the process of fitting people to places.

METHODOLOGY

Findings are derived from two sets of informants: a small sample of housing admission personnel and older adults meeting in focus group discussions. The goal of contact with both groups was to determine the information that is needed to effect appropriate matches between those needing housing and those who provide it.

Sample Selection

Housing providers were randomly selected from state and local lists of providers in central Maryland. Efforts were made to reflect diversity in size, location and level of care provided in the facilities selected. The final sample included respondents from 8 nursing homes, 2 group assisted housing settings, 4 domiciliary care homes, 2 small board and care homes, 3 senior apartment complexes and 1 continuing care retirement community (N = 20). The number of residents in these facilities ranged from three, in a small board and care home, to over a thousand in the continuing care retirement community. The median size was 58 residents. Staff sizes ranged from 1 to 800, with a median of 50. Five of the facilities described themselves as full, ten reported a waiting list, and five had vacancies at the time of the interview. Sixty percent (12) of the homes or facilities described themselves as having an affiliation with a religious group or hospital and half described themselves as nonprofit.

Older Consumers. Three focus groups, with 7-9 participants each, were held in the summer of 1992. Older adults were solicited from two Senior Centers. One was suburban, mostly white and middle-class. The other was an urban multi-purpose center which drew an ethnically and economically diverse clientele. Focus groups were recruited from the general Senior Center population, with efforts to ensure diversity in age, gender and race. Preference was given to individuals who were able to communicate clearly.

Most participants were female (63.6%), ages 65-74 (54.5%), lived in their own homes (68.2%), considered themselves retired (72.7%) and were white (54.5%). Ages ranged from the mid fifties to over 80, and a significant minority (40.9%) reported some financial strain ("Can't make ends meet" or "Sometimes can't afford what I need").

Procedures

Housing Providers. The person designated as responsible for admission in the home or facility served as the respondent to a structured, 15-minute telephone interview. A series of questions were asked about how people find out about their services, who contacts them to get information, the questions callers (both consumers and professionals) ask, important unasked questions, and their questions to potential clients.

Focus Groups. Focus group discussions were oriented around three hypothetical scenarios, where older adults needed to locate housing or evaluate alternative sites. The scenarios were employed to distance participants from the potential threat of discussing their own relocation (Morgan, 1988) and to obviate the need for specific experience. Large-type copies of the scenarios were distributed to visually-able participants, with participants encouraged to think about and write down their responses to the scenario. The two-hour sessions were audiotaped, with the tapes subsequently transcribed for analysis.

FINDINGS

Findings are presented in connection with particular questions, which were sometimes addressed by both and other times by only one of our samples.

Who Do Consumers Contact?

According to focus group respondents, most people don't know what to do when an older person needs to relocate to more supportive housing. According to a member of the first group, ". . . they learn after the situation happens." Another participant responded, "As to who to call, I would call various agencies because I am not really familiar myself with the various agencies so I would have to make a note to check the blue pages of the telephone directory . . ."

The focus group participants had a variety of ideas (N = 30 after removing within group redundancies) about who to contact to get information or referrals to housing. The ideas ran the gamut from clearly appropriate and specific (Information and Referral staff at a Senior Center) to not very appropriate (fire department, local politicians). Several of the recommendations were nonspecific, such as the statement to seek "a social worker," "the government," "an agency that does counseling."

There were three general types of responses: those that were specific and targeted, those using informal networks, and shots in the dark that might provide some helpful information.

Included among the specific and targeted responses were several likely to lead to fairly quick results (e.g., City Housing Department, local AAA, State Office on Aging, Senior Center, Social Worker, Nursing Home). Eleven responses were of the specific-targeted type. Four of the responses related to informal network resources (e.g., friends living in senior housing, friends, people from church, family members). These individuals would, in turn, be expected to provide information to begin the search in appropriate agencies.

The bulk of the remaining responses (N = 15) were individuals and groups who may direct the consumer to a specific source of housing information. Some (e.g., physician, fraternal organizations [some of which operate homes]) were more directly appropriate than others (e.g., schools, lawyers, area politicians, local police, employer, or union representative). Like the informal sources, these shots in the dark would probably yield a name or a telephone number to continue the search in a more targeted fashion.

It is clear that many individuals involved in the focus groups do not have a clear idea of how they should proceed to gather housing information. Many participants in our focus groups would contact inappropriate sources that would subsequently refer them on to others, in a potentially lengthy and stressful search process.

Who Contacts Providers?

Housing providers were also asked about the process by which potential residents contacted and gathered information from them. In response to, "How do most of your clients/residents find out about your services?" providers could select from nine structured answers or add others (median number of responses was 2). As results in Table 1 show, housing providers rely heavily on being known in the community and among professionals likely to make referrals, in addition to advertising, to make the community aware of their services. It appears that, from the providers' perspective, agencies are not among the major sources of referral.

When asked, "Who most often contacts you to get information on living here and the kinds of people you take?" frequent responses included the older person or couple, followed by a social worker, relatives, and physicians. Among the second and third most common contacts, relatives were most often mentioned (70%), followed by social workers (45%), physicians (20%), the older person or couple (15%), other professionals (10%) and nurses, friends and neighbors, and other (5% each). Clearly, from the view of the providers we interviewed, many of their informational contacts are made directly by the older person or close kin, followed by social workers.

TABLE 1. How Clients/Residents Find Out About Providers' Housing Services

	%	N
Generally Known in Community	65%	(13)
Other Professionals (e.g., Social Workers)	45%	(9)
Physicians or Nurses	40%	(8)
Advertisements	40%	(8)
Government Agencies (e.g., Office on Aging)	20%	(4)
From Friends, Neighbors	15%	(3)
Community Outreach Efforts	10%	(2)
Open-Ended Responses:		
Churches	5%	(1)

What Information Is Needed?

Both the provider sample and the consumers were asked to identify the information needed or used to determine the appropriateness and acceptability of particular housing options. Multiple responses to "questions . . . potential residents and their families typically ask you . . . to decide if (your facility) is an appropriate place for them?" are outlined in Table 2 (average 3-4 responses per provider).

Not surprisingly, the most asked consumer question is the cost of the facility, followed by the type of medical supervision, recreational activities, availability of financial supports, meal service, and current space availability. A number of issues expected to be important, such as room configuration, staff size and characteristics, and visiting hours, were reported by few providers as "typically asked."

Table 2 also summarizes the housing providers' responses to a parallel item on most asked questions by professionals (e.g., social workers or nurses) seeking housing for clients (average number of responses = 3). The focus for the professionals is markedly different from that of families. Only one provider said that professionals asked about costs, compared to 80% of elders and their family members. More professionals asked about medical supervision, and 90% of providers said that professionals asked about current space availability. Similarly 35% of providers said professionals asked about

TABLE 2. Questions Usually Asked by Potential Residents and Professionals

	Residents		Profs.	
Basic Costs of Housing/Services	80%	(16)	5%	(1)
Medical Supervision of Residents	55%	(11)	70%	(14)
Recreational Activities/Services	40%	(8)	10%	(2)
Subsidies/Financial Supports	30%	(6)	15%	(3)
Meal Service (Number/Types Provided)	30%	(6)	20%	(6)
Whether Space Is Available Now	30%	(6)	90%	(18)
Provision of Basic Services	20%	(4)	10%	(2)
Transportation Services	15%	(3)	15%	(3)
Therapeutic Services	15%	(3)	20%	(4)
Location	10%	(2)	10%	(5)
Extra Expenses	5%	(1)	0%	(0)
Room Size/Configuration	5%	(1)	0%	(0)
Special Diets	5%	(1)	0%	(0)
Visiting Hours/Limitations	5%	(1)	0%	(0)
Special Needs (e.g., Incontinence)	0%	(0)	35%	(7)
Single vs. Shared Rooms	0%	(0)	5%	(1)
Other Services	0%	(0)	10%	(2)
Staff Size	0%	(0)	5%	(1)
Open-Ended Responses:				
Security	15%	(3)		
Reputation	5%	(1)		
Allow Personal Possessions	5%	(1)		
Appearance of Unit	5%	(1)		

care of clients with special needs, (i.e., incontinent or bedfast), while none reported families asking such questions.

Given the fact that individuals seeking supportive housing may not know of the appropriate questions to ask, our housing providers were also asked to list up to three, ". . . questions or pieces of information do most families *neglect* to ask that you see as important?" Table 3 displays the cumulated, multiple responses to the question.

Most providers (85%) mentioned at least one, and nearly half mentioned two or more such questions. Meal service was the ne-

TABLE 3. What Important Information Do Families Neglect to Ask?

	%	N
Meal Service (Number and Types of Meals Provided)	25%	(5)
Medical Supervision of Residents	15%	(3)
Recreational Activities/Services	15%	(3)
Provision of Basic Services (Cleaning, Laundry)	15%	(3)
Special Needs (e.g., Incontinence, Wandering, Bedfast)	15%	(3)
Transportation Services	10%	(2)
Room Size/Configuration	10%	(2)
Visiting Hours/Limitations	10%	(2)
Basic Costs of Housing/Services	5%	(1)
Availability of Subsidies/Financial Supports	5%	(1)
Extra Expenses	5%	(1)
Special Diets	5%	(1)
Other Services	5%	(1)
Staff Size	5%	(1)
Staff Characteristics (Race/Training)	5%	(1)

glected item for one quarter of providers, while medical supervision, recreational activities, availability of services, and capacity to care for special needs were mentioned by three housing providers each. Housing providers, having experienced difficulties with poor person/environment fit in the past, may be more sensitive to some issues, such as special needs or meals, that are likely to create difficulties for a new resident.

Table 4 outlines questions that the housing providers typically ask to determine the appropriateness of a potential client for their supportive housing unit. Responses were cumulated in the table, and three responses were given by the average provider.

Clearly the items asked about by most providers focus in two areas–the medical condition of the potential resident and ability to pay. The responses reflect the providers' core orientations to health limitations and ADL/IADL status, ambulation, and medications, all of which would be significant determinants of their responsibilities should the individual move into that housing setting.

When we asked the focus groups, using two specific scenarios

TABLE 4. Providers' Questions of Potential Clients

	%	N
Health Status/Health Problems	85%	(17)
Ability to Pay	70%	(14)
ADL/IADL Status	55%	(11)
Ambulatory Status	35%	(7)
Medication Needs	25%	(5)
Social Needs	20%	(4)
Cognitive Status	20%	(4)
Behavior Problems	15%	(3)
Family Involvement	5%	(1)
Specialized Diet/Feeding	5%	(1)
Open-Ended Responses:		
Age	15%	(3)
Current Residence	10%	(2)
Expectations of Facility	5%	(1)
Past History	5%	(1)
Able to Handle Own Money	5%	(1)

(Mary, about to be released from the hospital after treatment for a broken hip, and John, no longer able to care for his wife with advancing Alzheimer's disease), to identify the issues about which information would be needed to make a housing choice, a wide variety of responses appeared.

All three groups prominently mentioned financial issues (e.g., cost of services, availability of subsidies, insurance or Medicare eligibility). In addition, all groups mentioned the number and types of services available (e.g., whether the home/facility provides meals, cleaning services, recreation, transportation, therapy, medication assistance, bed care, care for incontinence, etc.). Specific mention was made in two groups of staff size and medical staff (the presence of RN's or MD's on staff or on site). Also commonly mentioned were the staff qualifications to deal with clientele with special needs, prompted by the Alzheimer's disease scenario.

Other elements commonly mentioned across groups included visiting provisions, the location of the housing and its convenience to transportation for visitors or shopping, health care services, and the physical layout (stairs, room configurations and sharing). Two final issues that were common across groups were safety (fire, protection for those w/dementia, building and neighborhood security) and the availability of space or waiting list status.

Most of the remaining responses (four in group 1, 9 in group 2 and 7 in group 3) related to the quality of care in the housing environment. Quality of food and its adequacy, quality and qualifications of staff and management, attention to details in personal care, good attitudes of staff, a bright and cheerful environment, cleanliness, and a good reputation were examples. Quality of the environment was obviously a major concern to the focus group participants, and many shared stories of poor quality of care for relatives or friends.

DISCUSSION

In addition to the informational core of our focus group discussions, participants emphasized several key points in the process of housing selection. First, all groups reinforced the importance of matching housing to the level or type of impairment of the elder. "Do they have a staff there to give the services that they should." One cited the problem of persons who are "made an invalid before (their) time" by placement in too restrictive an environment.

Second, while recognizing the key role played by kin in this process, all three groups also emphasized maintaining the elder's input into the decision-making process as long as s/he was cognitively competent to do so. "I know in my case it (a discussion) would be very important. I would want to know what I was going to be faced with, because I would be the one moving." "Sit down and talk it over . . . This past weekend this is what we did–sit down and talk things over."

Third, a general concern was expressed about the lack of information people have about their alternatives and the difficulty of assessing various alternatives. "You go to these Senior places . . . and they'll tell you 'I'm sorry, we have a two year waiting list.' You have to go there in person and fill out an application and then it has to be so much of your income and all this and that before they'll decide if they'll take you." Long waiting lists, lack of affordable alternatives and the confusion of dealing with the bureaucracy were apparent. Participants reported widespread misconceptions about the type of care available in nursing homes and other types of alternative housing. "A lot of people think that when you go into a nursing home you're in there until the day you die . . . Nursing homes can be very helpful in short, recuperating programs."

Fourth, participants also emphasized the importance of visiting a site, preferably unannounced, to learn what really goes on there. Since much of the discussion focused on quality of care issues, participants were concerned about how to truly assess quality. An unannounced visit, several suggested, could provide better information needed to assess quality.

Finally, two of the groups critiqued poor attitudes of those providing care in nursing homes–lack of attention and caring toward their charges and a mercenary approach to the job. "That man's (a friend) wife had to come there on the days that he couldn't bathe himself and bathe him to make sure he was washed . . . half of the aides won't do it. They didn't want to be bothered." Another participant's wife had been in a "good" nursing home, but he claimed, ". . . love is only on paper. People who work there work only for their money."

CONCLUSION

Some key conclusions can be derived from this pilot study. First, consumers, professionals and providers have different perspectives on the process of housing selection, reflective of their involvement. These perspectives should not be expected to coincide, but differences may lead to inadequate communication and interfere with the placement process. If professionals are most concerned about availability of space but consumers ask about costs of services, it suggests that clear and complete communication is a must to enhance the match between persons and environments and minimize the stress inherent in this process. Maximizing information available to consumers and education in what to look for in housing is essential. Unless the family asks about the details, it is unlikely that harried professionals seeking placements or housing providers, seeking appropriate clients, will do so.

The lack of sufficient information was apparent from the focus group sessions. Older adults who are involved in locating assistive housing for themselves or relatives and friends are not clear about the most appropriate sources to call to gain the information they need. Many from our focus groups would be involved in lengthy searches to locate the housing should the need arise.

Clearly our focus group participants knew some of the key questions to ask, but were unfamiliar with the eligibility rules and requirements under which providers operate and receive reimbursement. The process gives a daunting and negative impression to potential clients, who see rules and red tape only as barriers to their search.

REFERENCES

Ambrogi, D. M. (1991). Nursing home admissions: Problematic process and agreements. *Generations, 14*, 72-74.

Anderson, E. A., Chen, A. & Hula, R. C. (1984). Housing strategies for the elderly: Beyond the ecological model. *Journal of Housing for the Elderly, 2*, 47-59.

Barker, J. C., Mitteness, L. S. & Wood, S. J. (1988). Gatekeeping: Residential managers and elderly tenants. *The Gerontologist, 28*, 610-619.

Beland, F. (1984). The decision of elderly persons to leave their homes. *The Gerontologist, 24*, 179-185.

Bernstein, J. (1982). Who leaves–who stays: Residency policy in housing for the elderly. *The Gerontologist, 22*, 305-313.

Betts, J., Moore, S. L. & Reynolds, P. (1981). A checklist for selecting board-and-care homes for chronic patients. *Hospital and Community Psychiatry, 32*, 498-500.

Butler, A., Oldman, C. & Greve, J. (1983). *Sheltered housing for the elderly: Policy, practice and the consumer.* London: George Allen & Unwin.

Daily, L. (1987). Housing options for the elderly. In J.A. Hancock (Ed.), *Housing the elderly* (pp. 227-244). New Brunswick, NJ: Center for Urban Policy Research.

Ehrlich, P. (1986). Hotels, rooming houses, shared housing and other housing options for the marginal elderly. In R. J. Newcomer, M. P. Lawton & T. O. Byerts (Eds.), *Housing an aging society: Issues, alternatives, and policy* (pp. 189-199). New York: Van Nostrand Reinhold.

Heumann, L. F. (1988). Assisting the frail elderly living in subsidized housing for the independent elderly: A profile of the management and its support priorities. *The Gerontologist, 28*, 625-631.

Huff, J. O. (1986). Geographic regularities in residential search behavior. *Annals of the Association of American Geographers, 76*, 208-227.

Kahana, E. (1974). Matching environments to needs of the aged: A conceptual model. In J. F. Gubrium (Ed.), *Later life: Communities and environmental policy.* Springfield, IL: Charles C Thomas.

Kelen, J. & Griffiths, H. A. (1983). Housing for the aged: New roles for social work. *International Journal of Aging and Human Development, 16,* 25-133.

King, S. & Collins, C. (1990). With a little help from my friends: Alzheimer's caregivers search for community services. Paper presented at the Annual Meeting of the Gerontological Society of America, Boston, November.

Lawton, M. P. (1980). *Environment and aging.* Monterey, CA: Brooks/Cole.

Lawton, M. P. (1985). The relevance of impairments to age targeting of housing assistance. *The Gerontologist, 25,* 31-34.

Mansbach, W. E. (1988). An analysis of elderly relocation and decision making processes. Unpublished Ph.D. Dissertation, University of Maryland, College Park.

Morgan, D. L. (1988). *Focus groups: Theory and practice.* Belmont, CA: Sage Publications.

Pynoos, J. (1987). Setting the elderly housing agenda. In Hancock, J. A. (Ed.), *Housing the elderly* (pp. 209-226). New Brunswick, NJ: Center for Urban Policy Research.

Rabin, D. L. & Stockton, P. (1987). *Long-term care for the elderly: A factbook.* New York: Oxford University Press.

Sherman, S. R. (1971). The choice of retirement housing among the well-elderly. *Aging and Human Development, 2,* 118-138.

Sherman, S. R. & Newman, E. S. (1979). Role of the caseworker in adult foster care. *Social Work, 24,* 324-328.

Sherwood, S., Morris, J. N. & Barnhart, E. (1975). Developing a system for assigning individuals into an appropriate residential setting. *Journal of Gerontology, 30,* 331-342.

Sherwood, S., Morris, J. N. & Sherwood, C. C. (1986). Supportive living arrangements and their consequences. In R. J. Newcomer, M. P. Lawton & T. O. Byerts (Eds.), *Housing an aging society: Issues, alternatives, and policy* (pp. 104-115). New York: Van Nostrand Reinhold.

Chapter 5

State Units on Aging
and Housing for the Elderly:
Current Roles and Future Implications

Phoebe S. Liebig

SUMMARY. One major goal of the Older Americans Act (OAA) is to promote suitable housing for the elderly through the aging network that includes the State Units on Aging (SUAs). Little is known, however, about SUA activity in this area. This article reports on the results of a recent survey of SUA housing efforts and roles played, collaborations and networks, resources, and priorities, accomplishments and future initiatives. To better link housing and services and expand housing options as some SUAs are already doing–especially in services coordination in existing housing, board and care, home equity conversion mortgages and assisted living–they must redefine housing as part of community-based care, vigorously focus political and advocacy skills on housing issues, and expand their capacity building and expertise in housing by resetting priorities and reallocating budgets.

Phoebe S. Liebig, PhD, is Assistant Professor of Gerontology and Public Administration, Andrus Gerontology Center, University of Southern California, Los Angeles, CA 90089-0191.

Research assistance from Deborah Brunner is gratefully acknowledged.

Partial research support was received from the U.S. Administration on Aging, Grant #90AT0386.

[Haworth co-indexing entry note]: "State Units on Aging and Housing for the Elderly: Current Roles and Future Implications." Liebig, Phoebe S. Co-published simultaneously in *Journal of Housing for the Elderly* (The Haworth Press, Inc.) Vol. 11, No. 2, 1995, pp. 67-84; and: *Housing Decisions for the Elderly: To Move or Not to Move* (ed: Leon A. Pastalan) The Haworth Press, Inc., 1995, pp. 67-84. Multiple copies of this article/chapter may be purchased from The Haworth Document Delivery Center [1-800-3-HAWORTH; 9:00 a.m. - 5:00 p.m. (EST)].

INTRODUCTION

Housing for the elderly has been an important policy issue for more than 30 years, predating the creation of many State Units on Aging (SUAs). In 1965, the Older Americans Act (OAA) was passed, serving as a catalyst for the creation of a national network of SUAs to serve persons age 60 and over. One of its eight goals was to promote "suitable housing, independently selected, designed and located with reference to special needs and available at costs which older citizens can afford" (PL 89-73). In subsequent amendments, the OAA emphasis on housing has been retained, with the Administration on Aging (AoA) using some of its funding to induce SUAs, Area Agencies on Aging (AAAs) and other organizations to increase suitable housing. Over the years, however, congressional mandates have tripled the mission of the aging network, but without a parallel increase in resources for housing or other OAA objectives, despite the growing numbers of older persons (Chelimsky, 1991; Gelfand & Bechill, 1991).

Housing for older Americans also has been a state policy objective (Schwartz, Ferlauto & Hoffman, 1991), in part influenced by national legislation but also by state-level concerns about the housing needs of older citizens. During the 1980s, state governments became more active in financing housing suitable for the aged, partly reflecting a decade-long trend in reduced federal funding for housing (Lammers & Liebig, 1990; Redfoot & Gaberlavage, 1991; Schwartz et al., 1991). SUA participation in this activity was not well documented; what little was known focused on examples of their practices in specific types of housing for the aged (see, for example, CSHA & NASUA, 1988; Struyk et al., 1989).

During this same period, it became increasingly clearer that suitable housing was not only a question of affordability and safety, but also of linkages to services for the impaired and frail elderly, so as to ensure "aging in place" (Tilson, 1990). The need for coordinating services with housing was raised at the 1981 White House Conference on Aging and became an issue for public and private funding sources, including the AoA, state governments and the Robert Wood Johnson Foundation.

In 1990, the enactment of the National Affordable Housing Act

(NAHA) authorized a number of programs benefiting older low-income owners and renters, many of which linked housing with services. Eligibility for federal funding required the development of five year plans by state and local governments that included the participation of social service agencies such as the SUAs and the AAAs, and a pooling of public and private resources, an activity also required of SUAs and AAAs by the OAA.

OAA objectives, recent shifts in federal and state housing policy for the aged, and the continued increase in the numbers of older persons make it likely that SUAs will be required to play more active roles in housing. These expectations will persist despite limited funding and the fact that housing policy is controlled by major players such as private developers, lending institutions, and other public sector agencies. To identify possible levels of future activity, it is necessary to understand current SUA efforts in housing, the subject of this article.

STUDY DESCRIPTION

Purposes

A survey of the SUAs was conducted in 1991 under the auspices of the AoA-funded Long-Term Care National Resource at UCLA/USC (LTCNRC). One purpose of this survey was to follow up on an earlier LTCNRC survey that focused on SUAs' then-current levels of effort and knowledge and possible future roles in eight areas related to long-term care, including home modifications and supportive housing (LTCNRC, 1989a). Other purposes were to obtain an accurate picture of recent SUA efforts in a variety of housing issues of increasing importance to long-term care and to expand on earlier studies, e.g., the 1988 joint report of the Council of State Housing Agencies (CSHA) and the National Association of State Units on Aging (NASUA), on usually low-level state initiatives in specific types of housing, such as home equity conversion mortgages (HECMs) and ECHO housing. A final purpose was to identify the capacity of SUAs to carry out and strengthen their housing endeavors in the future.

The study was designed to answer the following questions:

- To what extent are SUAs involved in housing issues and how does this involvement compare with earlier studies?
- With what groups do SUAs collaborate most frequently on housing issues and what are the results of these collaborations?
- What kinds of roles do SUAs characteristically play in housing for the elderly and what are the outcomes of those efforts?
- What kinds of resources (e.g., budget, staff number and expertise) do SUAs allocate to housing?
- What priority is assigned to housing and what housing initiatives have SUAs implemented in the past and will they implement in the future?

Data Collection

A survey instrument was developed, consisting of a ten-page questionnaire of 22 items of both closed-end and open-end questions. Advice on the design was provided by NASUA and the Council of State Community Affairs Agencies. Draft versions were critiqued by LTCNRC staff and the New Jersey SUA, as well as an outside consultant. The survey was mailed to 58 SUAs in April, 1991, with extensive follow-up telephone contacts conducted from mid-May through mid-September.

A total of 48 SUAs responded, for a response rate of 83 percent. Alaska, Colorado and Michigan declined to participate, while the seven other SUAs located in the Pacific and Caribbean islands did not respond to the initial or follow-up requests. No fewer than 44 SUAs responded to closed-end items.

RESULTS OF THE SURVEY
OF SUA HOUSING EFFORTS FOR THE ELDERLY

The results of the survey are presented below in five major sections: types of housing efforts; types of activity in housing and collaboration patterns in the past year; networks in housing issues; agency resources; and accomplishments, initiatives and priorities. The results provide an *overall* view of the SUAs, *as a group*, rather than singling out one SUA or groups of SUAs.

Types of Housing Efforts

The SUAs were asked to identify the year of their initial involvement in housing issues or programs; the amount of time spent on 20 different housing topics during the past three years; and the three issues to which most of their current efforts are devoted. The earliest year for SUA entry into housing-related issues was 1965, the year in which the OAA was passed; more than half (51 percent) entered into housing issues during the 1970s, with most (40 percent) doing so during the late 1970s, a period when OAA funding reached its peak (Chelimsky, 1991). A few SUAs initiated activity in housing only within the last four years.

During the past three years, SUAs have expended varying amounts of time on different housing issues, ranging from self-reported no time at all to a maximum amount. Table 1, "SUA Time Spent on Specific Housing Issues During the Past Three Years," reveals that *services coordination in existing housing, HECMs, board and care,* and *congregate housing, in that order,* have been the major SUA concerns. These areas were also identified as major SUA efforts in the 1988 CSHA & NASUA report. Naturally occurring retirement communities (NORCs), building codes, and single resident occupancy (SRO) hotels merited the least amount of SUA time during the past three years. Issues such as accessory apartments and ECHO housing, featured in the CSHA & NASUA report, were also among low effort areas. Several SUAs volunteered that they had been involved in issues such as design features of housing, mobile homes and training of housing managers.

SUA rankings indicated that the housing areas that are now most important are somewhat different from those of the past. Assisted living, services coordination in existing housing, and board and care are currently the three top SUA concerns. Other issues include foster care, shared housing and weatherization; nearly all reflect the current concern with housing options that combine housing with services.

Types of Recent SUA Activity in Housing, Collaborations

To obtain a more complete picture of recent activity, SUAs were asked to describe the level of their involvement in housing during the past year, by ranking a list of 10 activities, e.g., advocacy and

TABLE 1. SUA Time Spent on Specific Housing Issues During the Past Three Years
Ranked from High to Low (5–1)

Housing Issue	Mean
Services coordination in housing	3.24
Home equity conversion (HECs)	3.04
Board and care	2.96
Congregate housing	2.96
Assisted living	2.85
Home modification/repairs	2.78
Property tax rebates	2.70
Weatherization/energy conservation	2.69
Continuing care retirement communities (CCRCs)	2.60
Shared housing	2.57
Housing counseling	2.53
Foster care	2.20
Building retrofitting	2.13
Accessory apartments	2.09
ECHO housing	2.04
New purpose-built housing	2.02
Zoning	1.82
Single resident occupancy (SRO) housing	1.71
Building codes	1.59
Naturally occurring retirement communities (NORCs)	1.52

subcontracting, on a 5-point scale. As shown in Table 2, "Level of SUA Involvement in Housing in Past Year, by Type of Activity," the provision of housing information and referral *(I&R) for consumers* was the most frequent SUA activity, corroborating earlier studies (see CSHA & NASUA, 1988). Other recent SUA activity has revolved around *advocacy* and serving as a *convener of interested parties.* In the earlier LTCNRC survey (1989a), SUAs reported that they were most likely to exercise these two roles in the future in relation to home modifications and supportive housing; the activities least frequently engaged in–subcontracting and the creation of interagency agreements–were also identified as being less likely future roles (LTCNRC, 1989a). Some SUAs noted having been engaged in policy development, especially legislation and regulation, and in enhancing their AAAs' capacities in housing.

TABLE 2. Level of SUA Involvement in Housing in Past Year, by Type of Activity
Ranked from High to Low (5–1)

Type of SUA Activity	Mean
Information & referral: Consumers	3.52
Advocacy	3.30
Convener of interested parties	3.09
Coordinating services in existing housing	3.00
Technical assistance	2.80
Needs assessment/planning	2.76
Training	2.64
Information: Housing industry	2.54
Creating interagency agreements	2.40
Subcontracting	2.20

The SUAs were also asked to identify the types of activities in which they had been involved in the past year, relative to 20 specific housing issues (see Table 1 for the listing), and with whom. Because SUAs are expected to promote coordination within the aging network and with other organizations, they were asked to define whether their activities in each issue area involved AAAs alone, other agencies solely, or both.

SUA activities, in particular housing issues, vary greatly, as do their patterns of collaboration. In *consumer I&R,* SUAs focus most on HECMs and weatherization, followed by congregate housing, assisted living, and property tax rebates, generally working with AAAs alone. Nearly one-fourth work with AAAs alone in providing I&R on board and care, congregate housing and continuing care retirement communities (CCRCs), while more than 40 percent work with both AAAs and other organizations to educate consumers on home modifications/repairs (HMRs) and weatherization.

Advocacy efforts on services coordination in existing housing, congregate housing and assisted living were also important SUA activities recently, followed by weatherization, HECMs, property tax rebates, and board and care. In advocacy efforts, SUAs are more likely to work with all kinds of organizations. Approximately 40 percent worked with both AAAs and others to advocate for assisted living, HECMs, and weatherization, while between 25 to 30 percent collaborated with other organizations to promote CCRCs, board and care, and congregate housing.

In *convening interested parties,* SUAs brought groups together to address the issues of services coordination in existing housing, assisted living and congregate housing. They rarely convene only AAAs to address *any* housing issue. *Coordinating service provision* was another area of relatively high SUA activity, primarily in congregate housing and assisted living. SUAs work with both AAAs and other organizations: somewhat less than one-third on congregate housing and somewhat more than one in five on assisted living. These two housing issues were addressed across several types of activities: consumer I&R, advocacy, service provision in existing housing, and convening interested parties.

SUAs demonstrated middle-range activity in *technical assistance* (TA), working with both AAAs and other organizations in providing TA about services coordination in existing housing, congregate housing and HMRs, followed by HECMS and assisted living. *Needs assessment/planning* showed similar levels of activity, with very low levels of collaboration with AAAs alone; one in four SUAs reported working with both AAAs and other groups on services coordination.

Areas of low activity included *information to the housing industry,* usually on congregate housing and assisted living, in collaboration with non-AAAs. *Training* largely centered on HECMs and services coordination, with 20 to 24 percent of the SUAs involving both AAAs and other organizations. Areas of least activity included *creating interagency agreements* and *subcontracting.* When such agreements are forged, they center on services coordination, followed by congregate housing and HMRs, and involved both AAAs and other groups. SUAs provided minimal funds for nearly all housing areas; congregate housing, weatherization and assisted living were the major areas, involving AAAs and other organizations almost equally.

In all ten activities, SUAs did not work much with AAAs alone on housing issues. The highest rates of working with AAAs ranged from 11 to 22 percent, primarily in consumer I&R, TA and advocacy; only the topic of board and care received emphasis across these three types of activities. The low level of intrastate aging network collaboration on housing for the elderly is somewhat surprising, given the mandated roles of SUAs to develop state plans that meet OAA objectives.

By contrast, working arrangements with other organizations showed stronger patterns, with rates of collaboration ranging from 11 to 28 percent. The issues of congregate housing, CCRCs and new purpose-built housing were the content of advocacy, TA, and information to the housing industry. Collaborations with both AAAs and other organizations were especially pronounced, with high rates ranging from 20 to 44 percent. Services coordination in existing housing was the issue jointly addressed in eight activity areas. Assisted living and HECMs were also major issues on which SUAs worked with both AAAs and other groups, in at least five of the different types of activities. In the face of finite and sometimes shrinking resources and the major brokering roles required of SUAs, working with both kinds of organizations on any housing issue may be far more effective and efficient. SUAs' greater focus on non-AAA organizations may promote longer term impacts on the greater visibility of housing for the elderly within their respective states. This also can position them to develop the political and community support that is necessary for strengthening their capacity and performance (Hudson, 1986; Justice, 1988), also an objective of AoA's current National Eldercare Campaign.

To gain in-depth comprehension of SUA activities and their collaborations in the past year, a series of open-end questions was asked about six roles: advocacy, coordinating services, interagency agreements, subcontracting, technical assistance (TA), and training. SUAs were asked to describe briefly up to three specific activities, to whom those activities were directed, and their purpose and outcome; 45 responded to this section, but not all 45 SUAs responded to all six areas.

Advocacy related to housing was the role played most often by the SUAs; 39 reported a total of 81 advocacy efforts, which included giving testimony, providing information or training, and serving on committees. Characteristic targets were state legislatures, the aging network, other state departments (especially housing or housing finance), the governor, and county or other local agencies. The purposes of this advocacy usually were to initiate or to increase funding for some type of housing program, to promote awareness about housing for the elderly, and to affect rules and regulations. Outcomes included greater funding or fewer cuts in funding and increased awareness. For many, the outcome was still uncertain or pending.

Technical assistance (TA) was an important activity for 35 SUAs, with approximately half of them conducting at least two TA sessions, for a total of 58 efforts. TA generally took the form of training or on-site and other types of consultation, followed by work group formation, generation of statistics or research, and review/ analysis of documents. TA recipients were housing agencies, housing managers and developers/sponsors, AAAs, and state legislatures or other state departments. Purposes were to promote understanding of the housing needs of the aged, ensure the implementation of specific housing options (e.g., HECMs, personal care residences), and to design, market or monitor services. Outcomes varied greatly: more money allocated, an increase in assisted living options, more trained counselors and housing managers, and the development of proposal guidelines.

Coordinating service provision was described by 30 SUAs, for a total of 53 recent efforts, which included task force membership, the provision of grants, designation of a liaison person, TA, and training. Housing or housing finance agencies were the primary targets, followed by state social service or other kinds of human service departments, AAAs, HUD or the VA. The purpose was to reduce fragmentation, with the creation of better working relationships as the characteristic outcome.

Training was reported by 24 SUAs, with nearly half conducting three or more sessions, for a total of 55 efforts in the past year. Topics included housing options, services availability and access, normal aging, innovative housing, HECMs, tax rebates, and housing management skills. For the most part, training was conducted by conferences; nearly two-thirds of SUA training sessions were attended by 100 or more participants. The outcomes were better trained individuals and greater awareness about housing issues and options for the elderly.

A total of 23 SUAs reported 41 *subcontracting* activities in housing; eight SUAs awarded more than one subcontract, with two of them involved in four such activities. Dollars awarded ranged from slightly over $10,000 to $2.5 million; the majority (24) ranged from c. $10,000 to $100,000, while seven were for $1.5 to $2.5 million. Mentioned most often were awards to service providers, followed by housing agencies, consultants, developers, and housing finance authorities, primarily to develop congregate housing services demonstrations and HMR programs.

Creating interagency agreements was the role played least often; 23 SUAs reported a total of 36 such agreements. Eight had engaged in two or more agreements; nearly one-third reported involvement in developing a Comprehensive Housing Affordability Strategy (CHAS), a NAHA requirement. More than half of the agreements were formal Memoranda of Understanding (MOUs) or letters of agreement; the remainder were either informal or undesignated. The majority were negotiated with state housing, housing finance or other state departments. One-fourth were developed with HUD or the Farmers Home Administration (FmHA), the remainder with AAAs. The majority were vehicles for *future* action, e.g., planning, role and agenda definitions; thus, outcomes tended to be process-related, rather than programmatic.

Compared with earlier reports, there appear to be stronger SUA efforts in housing. Eleven reported having played all six roles during the past year, while another nine and seven SUAs had engaged in five and four roles, respectively. Thus 60 percent of the responding SUAs were involved in at least two-thirds of the six roles, a fairly high level of effort.

SUA Networks in Housing

SUAs are expected to mobilize a statewide commitment to the elderly; thus they were asked to rank on a 3-point scale their levels of interaction with a variety of organizations: aging and housing related federal agencies; state and local agencies offering a range of health, mental health and housing services; and non-governmental organizations in aging, health and housing.

Thirty percent of SUAs have frequent interaction with their AoA Regional Office, while one in seven interacts a good deal with the HUD Regional Office, and one in six with FmHA. In general, SUAs have *low* levels of contact with federal agencies on housing issues, in contrast with their high levels with other state level agencies. Half have frequent interactions with state social services agencies, which is consistent with their mandates to ensure the provision of comprehensive services for the elderly. (It should be noted that many SUAs are part of larger human services agencies.) Somewhat less than half (44 percent) work often with state community development and housing finance agencies, with smaller proportions contacting state health, mental health and rehabilitation service agencies about housing issues, as shown in Table 3, "Current SUA Priorities."

SUAs have less frequent contacts with local government agencies on housing issues compared to interactions with state agencies, but these contacts are still more numerous than those with federal agencies. More than four of every ten SUAs (43 percent) have frequent interactions with local adult protective services agencies. Just under one-third work often with local government health services and housing agencies.

With the exception of aging advocacy organizations, SUAs exhibit weak patterns of contact with non-governmental groups on housing issues. Fifty-seven percent have frequent contacts with groups such as AARP, with somewhat more than one-third reporting high levels of interaction with housing associations such as the

TABLE 3. Current SUA Priorities
Ranked from High to Low (1–8)

Priority Area	Mean
Community-based care systems development	1.48
Health services	3.64
Nutrition services	3.74
Transportation	4.17
Outreach	4.72
Housing issues and programs	5.48
Legal services	5.82
Mental health services	6.66

American Association of Homes for the Aged (AAHA), and somewhat more than one-quarter with home health associations.

In an open-end question, SUAs named the three agencies or
groups with which they had the most contact in the past year. The
agencies mentioned most often were housing or housing and community affairs (48 percent), housing finance (one-third), and AAAs
(25 percent). These levels of interaction indicate that SUAs are
incorporating these kinds of groups into their networks when ad-
dressing housing for the elderly.

Agency Resources

The survey sought to determine the general level of SUA budget
and personnel resources, as well as those specifically devoted to
housing efforts. As expected, total SUA budgets vary widely, ranging from a low of $100,000 to a high of $500,547,000 in the 1991
fiscal year. SUAs with the lowest budget levels have shown some
fluctuations over the past 3 years; the SUAs with larger budgets
have shown steady but incremental increases.

SUA housing-related budgets have also experienced some fluctuations over the past three years, from 0-33 percent in the current
year and from 0-27 percent in the two prior years. Overall, SUAs
devote *very* small proportions of their budgets to housing; *nearly 60
percent devote less than .5 percent of their current budget to housing.*

Fifty-five percent of SUAs reported receiving some funding
from state general revenues for housing, ranging from somewhat
more than $3,000 to $10 million. The second most frequent source
was Title III of the OAA, ranging from $9,800 to $748,000. Other
sources included AoA discretionary and other OAA funds and
Medicaid dollars, with a wide range of $1,100 to $30 million, and
other state funds.

SUAs reported a wide range in the numbers of paid staff from a
low of one to a high of 554, with staff paid to work on housing
issues ranging from none to seven, but larger SUAs do not necessarily have more housing staff. Nearly six of every ten SUAs have
less than one FTE in housing: 14 percent have 1/10 FTEs working
on housing, but 22 percent have two or more. Most (57 percent) do
not designate staff by a "housing" title, an indication that those

persons handle other matters. The majority of SUA personnel working on housing have been trained on the job or via attendance at professional meetings.

To gain expertise in housing, somewhat less than two-thirds (62 percent) use external consultants, usually on an unpaid basis. State housing agencies are the primary source (65 percent) of consultation for SUAs that use outside expertise, followed closely by federal housing agencies (55 percent) and their local counterparts (50 percent). Nearly one-third use housing developers or university personnel.

With few exceptions, SUAs devote minuscule amounts of their total budgets to housing issues. Moreover, the lack of staff assigned specifically to housing makes it difficult for them to develop expertise in this area. This situation is not likely to be rectified by the use of external consultants, especially if customary sources (i.e., public housing agencies) are constrained by their own budgetary problems.

ACCOMPLISHMENTS, FUTURE INITIATIVES, PRIORITIES

SUAs were asked to identify their three major accomplishments in housing during the past ten years, the three major housing efforts being considered or likely to be implemented in the next two to three years, and where housing fits into their priorities. The most important type of accomplishment was the creation of specific programs or model projects in housing; 41 were developed, with a major emphasis on HECMs, shared housing and congregate housing. Other accomplishments included policy development activities, data collection and planning, creation of housing networks, and consumer/residents' rights education.

The most common future initiative is to create or expand specific housing programs, with the increased coordination of supportive services in existing housing as the major goal. SUAs plan on developing new models of needs assessment, improving the delivery of services in congregate housing, and increasing services for elderly residents of publicly assisted housing, in keeping with their OAA mandates to serve the disadvantaged and the objectives of NAHA.

Other areas include consumer education; the creation or expansion of HECMs and HMRs, energy and security systems retrofit programs; training for housing managers, developers and AAA personnel; and new models of assisted living, small group or personal care homes. Capacity-building actions include developing comprehensive state-level planning, housing-related networks, a legislative agenda, and expertise in housing.

Despite these ambitions, the SUAs do not rank housing as an important priority; of eight areas, housing was ranked as number six, considerably outstripped by community-based care systems, health and nutrition services. As some respondents observed, however, it will not be possible to deliver quality community-based services to frail older persons if their housing is inadequate or unsuitable for the delivery of needed services.

CONCLUSIONS AND IMPLICATIONS FOR THE FUTURE

Most SUAs reported that they have been engaged in housing issues for the last ten years, usually in the areas of service coordination, HECMs, board and care, and congregate housing in the past three, with some more recent emphasis on assisted living and other housing options that are combined with services. While more SUAs appear to be involved in housing compared with earlier studies, not even one housing issue commanded a good deal of time and effort on the part of all or nearly all SUAs.

Levels of involvement in different types of activity also were low. Collaborations tended to involve both AAAs and other organizations, regardless of the type of activity undertaken or housing issue addressed, but by fewer than half of all SUAs. Consumer I&R and advocacy were the top SUA activities, with the latter targeted on elected policy makers and other state (especially housing and housing finance) agencies. But despite a strong pattern of networking with other state agencies, most SUAs do not create ongoing agreements that would enable them to secure more resources (i.e., budget, staff, political support) to help expand their efforts in housing.

The most frequent sources of SUA housing-related funds are state general revenues and Title III of the OAA. But total dollars allocated to housing are minuscule and staff with expertise or adequate training in housing are often lacking, a deficit that cannot be overcome by the use of consultants. With the federal budget deficit, OAA funding will be increased only marginally and the recent OAA reauthorization requires a focus on services for residents of federally assisted housing, foreclosure and eviction assistance, and a housing ombudsman program, among other mandates. State fiscal problems will likely preclude any major allocation of general revenues to housing for the aged, unless there is aggressive advocacy of the kind revealed by some SUAs in this study.

To meet the challenges ahead, all SUAs will need to focus on four areas: making housing a higher priority, exercising a higher level of organizational and political skills, positioning themselves to take advantage of new or less traditional sources of funding (e.g., NAHA), and expanding their capacity building. As the SUAs face the dilemma of doing even more with less for larger numbers of older Americans, they must reconceptualize their thinking about housing issues and programs. Community-based care systems–the number one SUA priority–are incomplete if housing is not seen as an integral component. SUAs and the aging network cannot develop comprehensive care systems if the housing of frail older persons is inadequate or unsuitable for optimal levels of functioning and the delivery of needed services. SUAs will need to reset their priorities and reallocate existing resources to ensure this; some are already doing so, as revealed in this study.

These readjustments in priorities will require strong advocacy for housing at state and federal levels by SUAs, using the impetus of the 1990 federal legislation (NAHA), and building the widespread political support to which elected officials respond. With the passage of NAHA, greater responsibility for effecting changes in housing priorities lies at the state and local level (Nelson & Khadduri, 1992). SUA policy development activities must marshall the continued support of traditional aging organizations including the AAAs and aging advocacy groups, but also the involvement of other major players in housing that have yet to play significant roles in aging issues (e.g., lending institutions). Given the ability of some SUAs, as shown in this survey, to build housing coalitions and exercise leadership in this regard, there is reason for guarded optimism about the success of more forceful advocacy for housing in the future.

In addition, SUAs need to explore vigorously other funding possibilities. Heavy dependence on OAA funds has often obviated the need for this kind of action (Hudson, 1986), and probably has made state policy makers less inclined to allocate additional resources, beyond any required match. New sources, such as NAHA, need to be tapped by SUAs to capture some additional resources for HECMs, home repairs and rural housing. In addition, greater SUA involvement in NAHA planning—the extent of which is an area for future research—will enable them to negotiate and coordinate statewide plans more efficaciously.

Finally, all SUAs must focus on their capacity building to meet the challenges of changed intergovernmental relations (Brown, 1983; Hudson, 1986; Justice, 1988), by improving their expertise and ability to anticipate changing circumstances as they affect housing for the elderly. In this survey SUAs indicated their need for greater information about federal and state housing legislation and about model programs and how to create them. The AoA is not in a strong position to provide this on its own (Chelimsky, 1991), so the SUAs must turn to AoA funded entities such as NASUA and the National Eldercare Institute for Housing and Supportive Services. SUAs must also use these and other state and regional resources to enhance their staff expertise in such areas as the attributes of successful models, the creation of viable housing coalitions, and the intricacies of housing finance and management.

As revealed in this study, some SUAs have developed the necessary expertise, primarily those with more years of experience in housing; however, even those with relatively recent entry into housing issues reported that they have moved rapidly into this area. It is clear that SUAs must balance off investments in capacity building in housing against the need to ensure the current delivery of services, an issue which is by no means new (see Brown, 1983; Hudson, 1986; Justice, 1988). Current political and budgetary climates require this kind of commitment to strategic planning. Without it, SUAs will not be able to meet the current or future housing and service needs of the elderly adequately.

REFERENCES

Brown, D.K. (1983). Administering aging programs in a federal system. In Browne, W.P. & Olson, L.X. (Eds), *Aging and public policy* (pp. 201-218). Philadelphia: Temple University.

Chelimsky, E. (1991). *The Administration on Aging: Harmonizing growing demands and shrinking resources.* Washington, DC: US Government Accounting Office (GAO/T-PEMD-91-9).

Council of State Housing Agencies & National Association of State Units on Aging (1988). *State initiatives in elderly housing.* Washington, DC: CSHA & NASUA.

Gelfand, D.E. & Bechill, W. (1991). The evolution of the Older Americans Act: A 25-year review of legislative changes. *Generations 15* (3): 19-22.

Hudson, R.B. (1986). Capacity building in an intergovernmental context: The case of the aging network. In Honadle, B.W. & Howith, A.M. (Eds), *Perspectives on management capacity building* (pp. 312-333). Albany, NY: SUNY Press.

Justice, D. (1988). *Long term care reform in six states.* Washington, DC: National Governors Association.

Lammers, W.W. & Liebig, P.S. (1990). State health policies, federalism, and the elderly. *Publius 20* (3): 131-140.

Long Term Care National Resource Center at UCLA/USC (1989a). *State units on aging: Current practices and future roles in long term care.* Los Angeles: LTCNRC.

Long Term Care National Resource Center at UCLA/USC (1989b). *Summary and analysis of Administration on Aging grant awards in supportive housing.* Los Angeles: LTCNRC.

Nelson, K.P. & Khadduri, J. (1992). To whom should limited housing resources be directed? *Housing Policy Debate 3*: 1-55.

Redfoot, D. & Gaberlavage, G. (1991). Housing for older Americans: Sustaining the dream. *Generations 15* (3): 35-38.

Schwartz, D.C., Ferlauto, R.C. & Hoffman, D.N. (1991). *A new housing policy for America: Recapturing the American dream.* Philadelphia: Temple University Press.

Tilson, D. (Ed), (1990). *Aging in place: Supporting the frail elderly in residential environments.* Glenview, IL: Scott, Foresman & Co.

Chapter 6

Factors That Influence Pre-Retirees' Propensity to Move at Retirement

Karen J. A. Johnson-Carroll
Jeanette A. Brandt
Joan R. McFadden

SUMMARY. The purpose of this study was to analyze the relative contributions of factors influencing preference to move upon retirement. Preference to move led to the propensity to move. Years in community, tenure preference upon retirement, opinion of size of house for retirement and existence of plans on where to retire led to both preference to move and propensity to move: structure preference led to preference to move. Maintenance skills led to the lessening of the propensity to move, and house size and age of respondent had a direct relationship to preference to move.

Karen J. A. Johnson-Carroll is Assistant Professor in Consumer and Family Studies, School of Education, San Francisco State University. Jeanette A. Brandt is Associate Professor in Apparel, Interiors, Housing & Merchandising, College of Home Economics, Oregon State University. Joan R. McFadden is Professor in Home Economics and Consumer Education, College of Family Life, Utah State University.

Data analyzed for this study are part of Regional Project W-176 "Housing and Locational Decisions of the Maturing Population: Opportunities for the Western Region." Financial resources for the collection of the data were provided, in part, by the U.S.D.A. Cooperative States Research Service.

[Haworth co-indexing entry note]: "Factors That Influence Pre-Retirees' Propensity to Move at Retirement." Johnson-Carroll, Karen J. A., Jeanette A. Brandt, and Joan R. McFadden. Co-published simultaneously in *Journal of Housing for the Elderly* (The Haworth Press, Inc.) Vol. 11, No. 2, 1995, pp. 85-105; and: *Housing Decisions for the Elderly: To Move or Not to Move* (ed: Leon A. Pastalan) The Haworth Press, Inc., 1995, pp. 85-105. Multiple copies of this article/chapter may be purchased from The Haworth Document Delivery Center [1-800-3-HAWORTH; 9:00 a.m. - 5:00 p.m. (EST)].

INTRODUCTION

The purpose of this study was to analyze the relative contributions of factors influencing preference to move upon retirement. This was accomplished using path analysis. Coveney and Rudd (1986) hypothesized and tested a causal model based on the Morris and Winter (1978) theory of housing adjustment to examine some determinants of housing satisfaction of rural, low-income, male family heads of work-force age. Their model had three levels: socio-demographic characteristics treated as exogenous variables, deficits or stressors as intervening variables and housing satisfaction as the endogenous variable. They measured household heads' maintenance skills as a socio-demographic variable, and viewed these maintenance skills as human resources able to be used to improve housing conditions.

Coveney and Rudd found that perceived low levels of maintenance quality decreased satisfaction, and that maintenance quality decreased with age of the head and increased with higher levels of maintenance skill of the head. In addition, they found that home ownership reduced maintenance needs but had little or no direct effect on housing satisfaction, and household characteristics tended to have an indirect effect on housing satisfaction.

HYPOTHESIZED MODEL

Based on Coveney and Rudd's (1986) model, this study's hypothesized model (see Figure 1) has been changed and refined to examine pre-retirees' perception of satisfaction with their home as measured by their current home for retirement usage, and their preference to move upon retirement. In addition, a fourth level was added, the propensity to move, as measured by the respondents' perception of the likelihood of the mobility decision. The objectives of this study were to see if the better the current status of the pre-retirees, the less likely would be the preference to move, and if the more the current housing is seen as appropriate for retirement, the less likely would be the preference to move.

FIGURE 1. Proposed Model of Factors That Influence Pre-Retirees' Propensity to Move at Retirement

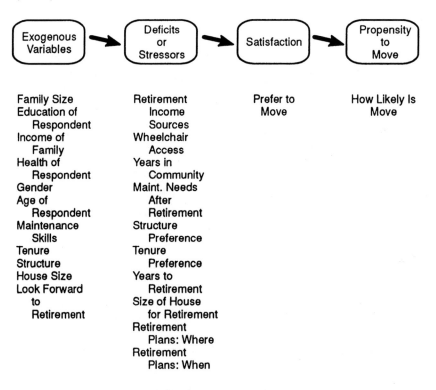

Exogenous Variables	Deficits or Stressors	Satisfaction	Propensity to Move
Family Size	Retirement	Prefer to	How Likely Is
Education of	Income	Move	Move
Respondent	Sources		
Income of	Wheelchair		
Family	Access		
Health of	Years in		
Respondent	Community		
Gender	Maint. Needs		
Age of	After		
Respondent	Retirement		
Maintenance	Structure		
Skills	Preference		
Tenure	Tenure		
Structure	Preference		
House Size	Years to		
Look Forward	Retirement		
to	Size of House		
Retirement	for Retirement		
	Retirement		
	Plans: Where		
	Retirement		
	Plans: When		

DESCRIPTION AND DEFINITION OF MODEL'S VARIABLES

Exogenous Variables

Coveney and Rudd's (1986) model used few of Morris and Winter's (1975) socio-demographic variables, as there was a lack of variation in their sample. As this study used respondents from an age-stratified random sample, additional socio-demographic variables have been added to the model developed by Coveney and Rudd.

Family size. Size of family can alter the financial well-being of people during retirement. Dual earner households and reduced number of children increase the ability of the elderly to achieve financial well-being (Easterlin, Macdonald, & Macunovich, 1990). Brandt, McFadden and Malroutuk (in press) found that single person households are more at risk than others during retirement and need to be targeted for retirement planning. Indeed, in 1988, 60% of elderly women lived alone, and elderly women have a substantially higher poverty rate than others (Hurd, 1990). Measurement of family size in this study measures the total number of people living in the respondent's home.

Education. Coveney and Rudd (1986) found that education of very low-income male heads of households had little direct or indirect effect on housing satisfaction except for the education needed to gain maintenance skills. However, Brandt et al. (in press) noted that the education level of pre-retirees explains some variability on the number of sources of planned retirement income. Reid and Zeigler (1980) hypothesize that the more rewarding jobs in terms of income and prestige (which affect retirement income and plans) are because the workers are more highly educated. Cramer et al. (1983) found that the higher the education, the larger the house size. Education in this study measures level of education of respondent from "less than 12 years" to "graduate or professional degree (doctoral)."

Income. Income of pre-retirees explained some variability in the number of sources of planned retirement income (Brandt et al., in press), and income is needed to finance moves and can be expected to positively affect the decision to migrate (Goss & Paul, 1986). An explanation of mobility after retirement arises from the need to alter living costs to family size and responsibilities (Lee, 1980). Hurd (1990) found that wealthier couples live longer than poorer couples (Hurd, 1990). The household income variable in this study measures total family income before taxes in 1989 from "less than $10,000" to "$95,000 or more."

Health of respondent. The health, both good and bad, of retirees has an effect on retirement plans (Prothero & Beach, 1984). Indeed, the health status of an individual can be a major factor in the decision to move. Poor health might inhibit migration, or because of poor health, a person might have to move to a healthier climate, or to obtain care (Patrick, 1980). The health variable is measured by the respondent choosing to describe their health from "excellent" to "poor."

Gender. In 1985 a 65-year-old woman could expect to live 4.1 years longer than a 65-year-old man. By 2080 this gap is expected to increase to 5.2 years, producing obvious effects on social security and pensions (Hurd, 1990). In addition, females are less likely to be homeowners, and more likely to live in smaller housing (Morris & Winter, 1978), reducing a source of possible equity. Analyzing the differences in retirement for males and females has some problems. For example, Belgrave (1989) found controversy when relating definitions of retirement to women, due to the variability of their work histories. Although retirement may have come after 40 years of employment for most men, this was not entirely true for women. Some older women who had been housewives for virtually their entire lives defined themselves as retired, yet some who had been employed full-time since their teens, not leaving the labor force until their sixties, referred to themselves as housewives. Some women defined their retirement status based on their husband's ties to the labor force, and others saw themselves as housewives regardless of their own work histories. Furthermore, women were considerably less likely than men to be fully retired. Fourteen percent of women aged 60-64 were found to have continued productive activity of either a paid or volunteer nature after retirement.

While both males and females felt themselves capable of physical tasks in the home (Morrison et al., 1978), females were less likely to fulfill plans for housing adjustment (Duncan & Newman, 1976). This could be because females have lower incomes and the lack of taught ability to do household repairs (Abdel-Ghany & Nickols, 1983: Glazer, 1983). Gender of respondent is a dichotomous variable–male and female.

Maintenance skills. Coveney and Rudd (1986) found that maintenance skills directly and indirectly impact housing satisfaction. This could be because the presence of someone who can do household repairs is one of the best predictors of the adoption of certain modifications in the home (Leonard-Barton, 1981), thus allowing the adoption of preferred alterations. Yet, while Coveney and Rudd found that maintenance skill may provide a better image of self and home, thus enhancing ratings of satisfaction independent of actual quality of housing, Goss and Paul (1986) found that the possession of a higher level of general skills (as measured by years of experience) actually increases mobility. Maintenance skill in this study was a mean score derived from how the respondent rated his/her own skill level at seven home maintenance tasks, choosing between "above average," "average," and "below average."

Age. The effect of age on mobility seems to vary. Rhodes (1983) found age to be the strongest and most consistent predictor of work-related behaviors, such as retirement. Age has been found to positively influence expectations of retirement and actual retirement plans (Prothero & Beach, 1984). Along with education and income, age explains 22.577% of the variability on the number of sources of planned retirement income (Brandt et al., in press). While Goss and Paul (1986) found that the older the person the less likely he/she will be to move, Patrick (1980) found that mobility appears to decline until middle age, then swing upward through retirement age until the 70's, and then decline again. Coveney and Rudd (1986) found the effect of age of the head of household on housing satisfaction was small due to the offsetting indirect influence of a higher maintenance need. Age of respondent in this study measures the respondent's age in the last ten months of 1989 or first two months of 1990.

Tenure. The tenure of a dwelling is linked to better household conditions, satisfaction and making more maintenance decisions (Johnson-Carroll, Brandt, & Olson, 1987). Renters are generally not expected to do as much maintenance and repair as owners (Coveney & Rudd, 1986; Eichner & Morris, 1984; Tyler, Lovingood, Bowen, & Tyler, 1982), probably because the tenants see that in some household adjustments the cost benefits go to the landlord, not themselves (Eichner & Morris, 1984). Tenure of dwelling in this study is a dichotomous variable–owners and renters.

Structure. Pickvance (1973) found that household characteristics are a major determinant of mobility. Low income families are more likely to live in rental units attached to other residences (Stern, Black, & Elworth, 1982). Measurement of structure in this study was a dichotomous variable–single family house detached from any other structure and any other type of structure.

House size. Coveney and Rudd (1986) found with their model that larger families tended to have fewer bedrooms than needed, which lowered housing satisfaction. Families that live in smaller dwellings tend to be low income families (Cramer et al., 1983; Tyler et al., 1982). House size in this study was measured by the number of square feet in the home and ranged from "less than 1,000 square feet" to "more than 2,000 square feet."

Respondent looking forward to retirement. Workers who have positive expectations about retiring are more likely to retire and are more likely to be satisfied with retirement than are those workers with negative expectations (Prothero & Beach, 1984). A low sense of self-efficacy in relation to retirement was linked to a lower degree of planfulness (for example, planning for retirement mobility) (Atchey, 1974). Migration movements upon retirement are highly specific in nature: toward the better life as defined in terms of the wants and abilities of the aged (Lee, 1980). Predisposition toward retirement in this study measures how respondent felt about his/her retirement, from looking forward to, feel somewhat neutral about, or did not look forward to retirement from active employment.

Intervening and Endogenous Variables

Retirement income sources. Economically advantaged retired households have been equated with those that have multiple retirement income sources (Brandt et al., in press; Kart, Longino, & Ullman, 1989). It has been found that full retirees have, on average, 46% of pre-retirement income if they receive one retirement benefit and 60% of pre-retirement income if they have more than one benefit (Grad, 1990). The retirement income sources variable in this study is measured by the respondent's indication of the number of sources of planned retirement income.

Wheelchair access. People often do not ask themselves whether or not their homes can accommodate a wheelchair until the need arises through an accident, illness or the aging process (McFadden, Brandt, & Tripple, 1989). Often, a home must be altered significantly to accommodate a wheelchair. To retirees, however, a change in dwelling structure can be viewed as upsetting. The house as it stands is a major source of security and comfort for some, while other retirees try to make their house as secure as possible for future needs (Wilk & Wilhite, 1983). Kilty and Behling (1985) found that planning one's resources (for example, planning for access in one's home) was positively related to fulfilling plans to retire. McFadden et al., (1989) hypothesize that in the future, people will choose homes that can be adapted to wheelchair use, and that it will be a common family decision to choose housing that is accessible and/or an adaptable home. Wheelchair access in this study measures to what extent the respondent feels his/her home could accommodate a person with a wheelchair in seven specific areas within the home.

Years in community. Many elderly prefer to remain where they have established friends and relatives (Lee, 1980) rather than move, and the longer a person has lived in a community, the less that person preferred to move upon retirement (Brandt, 1989). Gigy (1986) found in her study that a large percentage of retired women particularly emphasized the importance of having family and/or friends around them when they retired, and that these established networks were needed for a successful retirement. Another viewpoint could be that inertia is a major factor in mobility decisions. It is simpler to do nothing than to do something (Lee, 1980). Measurement of years lived in the community was based on the number of years the respondent lived in or near the community in which the home currently was located.

Maintenance needs after retirement. Maintenance need was one of two strongest influences on housing satisfaction (Coveney & Rudd, 1986). Dwellings the elderly lived in were often older and in need of repairs (Walden & Meeks, 1982). This could be because older residents may have health problems that prevent them from being able to maintain their home (Eichner & Morris, 1984). However, maintenance skill influences quality of maintenance whether or not the skilled person owns the home (Coveney & Rudd, 1986). Maintenance needs after retirement measures how the respondent plans on having seven home maintenance tasks done after retirement–by themselves, spouse/partner, friend/relation, or hired person.

Structure preference for retirement. Structure of a dwelling, particularly if perceived as a deficit, has been found to have an effect on the desire to move (Morris & Winter, 1978). Morris and Jakubczak (1988) found that perceived structure and tenure deficits had a direct influence on satisfaction, and a direct and indirect (through satisfaction) influence on the propensity to move. Baille (1990) found that housing type had both an indirect (through attractive neighborhood) effect and a direct effect on satisfaction, and both an indirect (through satisfaction) and a direct effect on intention to move. Dillman, Tremblay and Dillman (1979) found that respondents in the older age categories showed a preference for duplexes, apartments or mobile homes, while in contrast, Brandt (1989) found that persons approaching retirement preferred to own a single family detached dwelling. Structure preference in this study is a dichotomous variable–preference for a single family house detached from any other house, and any other type of housing structure.

Tenure preference for retirement. Tenure deficits have been found to have an effect on satisfaction and propensity to move (Morris & Jakubczak, 1988; Morris & Winter, 1978). Elderly often view expenditures on durable goods, such as housing, as yielding lower benefits for the long term and are less likely to make capital housing expenditures (Walden & Meeks, 1982). Dillman et al. (1979) found that while the preference for home ownership is strong among most age groups, regardless of current tenure status, respondents in the older age categories are most likely to prefer to rent a duplex, an apartment, or own a mobile home placed on rented space. They suggest that the norms for ownership are probably not as important to older people. Yet Brandt (1989) found that most persons approaching retirement preferred to own their home. Tenure preference in this study is a dichotomous variable–rent or own.

Years to retirement. The number of years before one retires can profoundly affect the way retirement and its decisions are viewed. Erdner and Guy (1990) found that both men and women had increasing problems with retirement when retirement was near. The loss of status and income was seen as particularly disturbing. Anson, Atonovsky, and Sagy (1989) found that the losses associated with retirement were major and were felt most keenly upon the verge of retirement. In her study of female retirees, Szinovacz (1986) found that some women preferred to postpone retirement regardless of health reasons or stable pre-retirement incomes. Women who are older and nearer to the actual time of retirement are more likely to retire at ages 62-64, but younger women are more likely to plan to retire either before 62 or at age 65 (Shaw, 1984).

Number of years to retirement was indicated by respondents and calculated by subtracting 1990.

Size of house for retirement. While size of house as particularly measured in number of bedrooms can be expected to influence housing satisfaction (Morris & Winter, 1978), an explanation for mobility after retirement arises in part from the need to adapt housing to family size and responsibilities (Lee, 1980). When children leave home, home-owning tends to fall off (Pickvance, 1973). The size of the house for retirement was measured by the respondents' opinion of whether their current home was too large, about the right size, or too small for use during retirement.

Retirement plans–when and where. It is often difficult to compare relative influences when considering whether to undertake a course of action, particularly when the action in question is complex and when it has potentially far reaching and profound implications for one's life (Prothero & Beach, 1984). It may seem obvious that the evaluation of what happens after retirement, evaluating current status and planning for retirement, affects actual retirement (Hurd, 1990), but financial status or economic conditions are influenced by items that include personal and/or family decisions during pre-retirement (Brandt et al., in press). Kilty and Behling (1985) found that planning for one's retirement (including decisions such as mobility) helped respondents actually follow through on their plans. Retirement planning for this study was divided into two areas: planning when to retire, and planning where to retire. Respondents were asked if they had planned where to retire, and/or when they would retire.

Satisfaction with current housing for retirement. Brand (1989) found in her study of housing and community preferences that most people approaching retirement preferred a dwelling in the same state or community where they currently lived. Prothero and Beach (1984), in their study of retirement plans and intentions, found that expectations of retirement and what would happen upon retirement, such as moving, were used to predict intentions of what would actually occur during retirement and 78% of these predictions occurred. The prediction of behavioral intentions is a necessary and sufficient condition for the prediction of a behavior (Ajzen & Fishbein, 1975), although this is not unconditionally true. Fishbein

(1967) and Wicker (1969) report that near perfect correlations between intentions and behavior result only when there is a specific intention and a specific situation. Satisfaction with the current home for retirement is measured in this study by whether the respondent preferred to move from the current community upon retirement or preferred to stay in the current community.

Propensity to move. Coveney and Rudd's (1986) model was expanded to include the propensity for a certain action, in this case the likelihood of actually moving. In Prother and Beach's (1984) study, intentions regarding retirement were used to predict actions and 76% of these predictions were correct. It has been found that desired mobility is more frequent than planned mobility, which in turn is more frequent than actual mobility (Van Arsdol, Sabagh & Butler, 1968). In this study, the propensity to move was measured by the respondents' perception of how likely they were to actually move after retirement.

PROCEDURES

The data used in this study were collected as part of a mail survey conducted by the Western Regional Agricultural Experiment Station Committee (W-176), "Housing and Locational Retirement Decisions: A Study of Pre-Retirees in Four States," during February and March, 1990. Data from the four states: Oregon, Utah, Michigan, and Idaho were analyzed. The sample was ordered from Survey Sampling Incorporated which drew a random sample of the population between 40 and 65 years of age. The overall response rate in the four states was 43%.

The respondents were most likely to be full-time employed males, with a median age in the range of 40-55 years, living in households of two persons who earned a total income of $35,000-$49,999. The education of respondents tended to be fairly evenly spread among "high school grad" (22.5%), "some college" (22.6%), and "Bachelors" (20.6%). Most respondents described their health as "excellent" (46.4%) or "good" (45.7%), and looked forward to retirement (53%). The homes of the respondents tended to be single family structures owned with a mortgage. Sizes of these structures were fairly evenly distributed between 1000-1500 sq. ft. (34.2%), 1501-2000 sq. ft. (30.7 %) and over 2000 sq. ft. (26.6%).

Path analysis provided the method by which quantitative estimates of the causal effects were estimated. Multiple regressions, which gave the beta weights, were conducted. The beta weights indicate how much change occurs in the endogenous variables, given that there is one unit of change in the exogenous variable and all other variables are held constant. Beta weights not meeting the criterion for significance (p < .01) were rejected.

RESULTS

The following paths are supported in the model (see Figure 2 and Tables 1 and 2).

Exogenous Variables

Only three exogenous variables: age of respondent, maintenance skill of respondent and current house size, had direct relationships (p < .01) to the last two variables in the model: preference to move, and propensity or how likely is move. The older the respondent, and the larger his/her home, the less likely was the respondent to prefer to move. The higher the maintenance skills of the respondent, the less likely was a move upon retirement.

Endogenous Variables

Five of the ten deficit or stressor variables, retirement income sources, wheelchair access, maintenance needs after retirement, years to retirement, and retirement plans: when, were found to be significantly related to one or more exogenous variables, but not to contribute significantly (p < .01) to the endogenous variables further along the model.

Education, current income, age and house size were significantly related to the number of retirement income sources, but retirement income sources was not significantly (p < .01) related to either preference to move or propensity to move. Family size was found to

FIGURE 2. Test Path Analysis Model with Significant (p < .01) Pathways

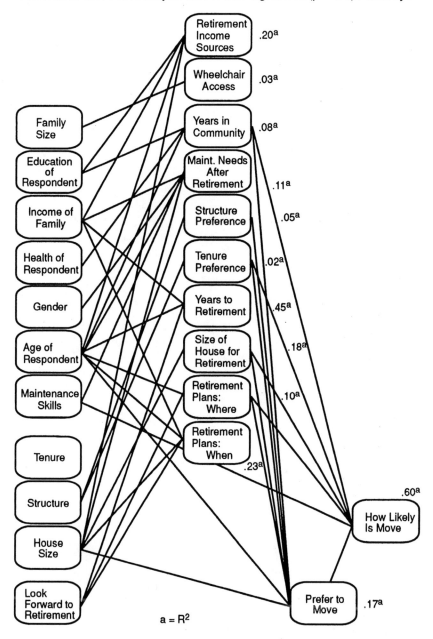

a = R²

TABLE 1. Resultant Betas of the Regression Analyses of Stressors/Deficits

	Ret. Income Sources		Wheelchair Access		Years in Community		Maintenance Needs		Where to Retire Plans	
	Sign.	Beta	Sign.	Beta	Sign.	Beta	Sign.	Beta	Sign.	Beta
Family size	.584	-.02	.012	.09*	.035	.07	.419	-.03	.414	.03
Education of Resp.	.000	.12*	.244	.04	.001	-.10*	.662	.01	.638	.01
Household Income	.000	.26*	.132	-.05	.484	.02	.000	.14*	.289	-.03
Health of Resp.	.030	-.06	.021	-.08	.000	.12*	.847	.01	.026	-.07
Gender of Resp.	.271	-.03	.370	.03	.804	.01	.000	-.17*	.255	.04
Maintenance Skills	.668	-.01	.061	-.06	.351	-.03	.000	.22*	.656	-.01
Age of Resp.	.001	.10*	.021	.08	.000	.20*	.005	-.09*	.000	.27*
Tenure (rent/own)	.880	.00	.255	.03	.776	-.01	.870	-.00	.041	-.06
Structure	.531	.02	.613	-.02	.271	.03	.576	-.02	.218	.04
House size	.000	.18*	.061	.06	.208	-.04	.000	.13*	.110	-.05
Look forward to retirement?	.086	-.05	.312	-.03	.141	-.04	.213	.04	.000	-.17*

	Structure Preference		Tenure Preference		Years to Retirement		House Size for Ret.		When to Retire Plans	
	Sign.	Beta	Sign.	Beta	Sign.	Beta	Sign.	Beta	Sign.	Beta
Family size	.515	.02	.213	.04	.199	.03	.079	-.06	.843	.00
Education of Resp.	.934	.00	.366	-.03	.174	.03	.882	-.00	.250	.03
Household Income	.162	-.05	.494	-.02	.000	-.20*	.424	-.02	.010	.08*
Health of Resp.	.517	-.02	.306	-.03	.223	-.03	.285	.03	.995	-.00
Gender of Resp.	.253	.04	.659	-.01	.119	.04	.969	-.00	.826	.00
Maintenance Skills	.112	-.05	.202	-.04	.870	.00	.694	-.01	.054	-.05
Age of Resp.	.034	-.07	.250	-.04	.000	-.60*	.102	-.05	.000	.24*
Tenure (rent/own)	.557	-.02	.483	.02	.110	-.04	.655	-.01	.619	.01
Structure	.000	.17*	.007	.09*	.511	.03	.029	-.06	.199	.04
House size	.124	.05	.565	.02	.405	.02	.000	-.37*	.000	-.11*
Look forward to retirement?	.451	-.02	.241	-.04	.000	.19*	.081	.05	.000	-.39*

* = p < .01

TABLE 2. Resultant Betas of the Regression Analyses of Preference to Move and How Likely Is Move

	Preference to Move		How Likely Is Move	
	Sign.	Beta	Sign.	Beta
Family size	.100	−.05	.057	−.04
Education of Resp.	.170	.04	.668	.01
Household Income	.164	.05	.133	−.04
Health of Resp.	.978	.00	.302	−.02
Gender of Resp.	.519	.02	.350	.02
Maintenance Skills	.530	.02	.001	−.07*
Age of Resp.	.000	−.15*	.030	−.06
Tenure (rent/own)	.297	.03	.782	−.01
Structure	.124	.05	.619	−.01
House size	.014	−.09*	.295	.03
Look forward to retirement?	.440	−.02	.490	.02
Ret. Income sources	.795	−.01	.537	.01
Wheelchair access	.129	−.04	.153	−.03
Years in community	.000	−.12*	.000	−.08*
Maintenance needs	.599	−.02	.583	−.01
Structure preference	.002	−.09*	.647	−.01
Tenure preference	.001	−.09*	.005	−.06*
Years to retirement	.023	−.09	.072	−.05
House size for ret.	.000	−.11*	.012	−.05*
Where to ret. plans	.000	−.27*	.000	−.09*
When to ret. plans	.061	.06	.096	.04
Preference to move			.000	.70*

* = p < .01

be related only to wheelchair access, and wheelchair access, too, was not found to contribute to the endogenous variables further along the model. Maintenance needs after retirement had significant (p < .01) relationships with household income, gender, maintenance skills and age of respondent, and house size, but not to other exogenous variables. The fourth stressor or deficit variable found not to contribute to the remaining levels of endogenous variables was years to retirement. However, years to retirement was found to be significantly (p < .01) related to household income, age of respondent, and how much the respondent looked forward to retirement. Whether the respondent planned when to retire was found to be related to household income, age of respondent, house size and whether the respondent looked forward to retirement, yet it too did not have a significant (p < .01) relationship with the endogenous variables further along the model.

Years in Community

Education, health, and age of respondent all had a significant relationship with the number of years in the community. The lower the level of education, the better the health, and the older the respondent, the more years were spent in the community. In addition, these three exogenous variables had an indirect effect on the preference to move and propensity to move variables, as the number of years in the community had a direct significant (p < .01) relationship with both, and in addition, indirect influence on propensity to move through preference to move. The longer a person spent in the community, the less was the preference to move, and the less was the propensity or likelihood of moving.

Structure and Tenure Preference

If the current household structure is a single family detached dwelling owned by the pre-retiree, then there is a significant (p < .01) possibility that the pre-retiree's structure/tenure preference for retirement is an owned/single family detached dwelling. In addition, current structure is indirectly related to preference to move upon retirement through retirement structure preference, and to propensity to move through preference to move. If retirement structure preference is an owned single family detached dwelling, then the preference to move is less, and the propensity or likelihood to move is less. In addition, tenure preference for retirement has a direct relationship with propensity to move. If the pre-retiree prefers an owned home, a move is less likely. Current tenure is not significantly (p < .01) related to any endogenous variables in this model.

Size of House for Retirement

The only exogenous variable to be significantly (p < .01) related to opinion of size of house for retirement is the size of the pre-retiree's current house. The larger the current house, the more the pre-retiree felt it was too large for retirement use. Opinion of size of house for retirement was also directly related to preference to move and propensity to move, and indirectly related to propensity to move through the preference variable. If the pre-retiree felt the house was too small for retirement use, there was less of a preference to move, and less of a likelihood to move.

Plans to Retire: Where

Planning where to retire was significantly (p < .01) related to the age of the respondents and how much they looked forward to retirement. The older the respondents, and the more they looked forward to retirement, the more likely they were to have plans of where to retire. In addition, existence of plans of where to retire was directly related to both preference to move and propensity to move. The more likely the respondents had plans where to retire, the less likely they were to prefer to move, and the less likely was their propensity to move.

SATISFACTION LEVEL

Preference to Move Upon Retirement

Preference to move upon retirement was significantly (p < .01) and strongly related to the propensity or the likelihood of moving. The stronger the preference to move, the more likely the pre-retirees felt they would move.

IMPLICATIONS

This study supports previous research studies which have found dissatisfaction with current housing to be the strongest determinant of propensity to move. In addition this study has shown that many variables which could be loosely considered as characteristics describing a life and retirement that closely adhere to society's norm lessen the preference and propensity to move upon retirement. Preference and propensity to move are less if pre-retirees are healthy, look forward to retirement, are confident of their maintenance skills, are older, live in a small house that is a detached single family dwelling, have spent many years in the same community, have definite tenure/structure preferences that mimic their current structure (only perhaps smaller), and definite plans where to retire.

REFERENCES

Abdel-Ghany, M. & Nickols, S.Y. (1983). Husband/wife differentials in household work time: The case of dual-earner families. *Home Economics Research Journal, 12*(2), 159-167.

Ajzen, I. & Fishbein, M. (1975). The prediction of behavior from attitudinal and normative variables. In A.E. Liska (Ed.), *The Consistency Controversy: Readings on the Impact of Attitude on Behavior.* New York: John Wiley & Sons.

Anson, O., Atonovsky, A., & Sagy, S. (1989). Family, gender, and attitudes toward retirement. *Sex Roles, 20,* 355-369.

Atchley, R. (1974). The meaning of retirement. *Journal of Communication, 24,* 97-101.

Baillie, S. (1990). Dwelling features as intervening variables in housing satisfaction and propensity to move. *Housing and Society, 17*(3), 1-15.

Belgrave, L. (1989). Understanding women's retirement. *Generations,* 49-52.

Brandt, J.A. (1989). Housing and community preferences: Will they change in retirement? *Family Economics Review, 2*(2), 7-11.

Brandt, J.A., McFadden, J.R. & Malroutuk, Y.L. (in press). Pre-retirees family structure: Impact on retirement. Unpublished manuscript. Oregon State University, Agricultural Research Center Project No. 9551.

Coveney, A.R. & Rudd, N.M. (1986). Determinants of housing satisfaction of low-income, rural, male family heads. *Housing and Society, 13*(1), 3-18.

Cramer, J.C., Dietz, T.M., Miller, N., Craig, P.P., Hackett, B.M., Kowalczyk, D., Levine, M., & Vine, E.L. (1983). The determinants of residential energy use: A physical-social causal model of summer electricity use. In B.M. Morrison and W. Kompton (Eds.), *Proceedings of Families and Energy Coping with Uncertainty* (pp. 595-616). East Lansing, MI: Michigan State University.

Dillman, D.A., Tremblay, Jr., K.R., & Dillman, J.J. (1979). Influence of housing norms and personal characteristics on stated housing preferences. *Housing and Society, 6*(1), 2-19.

Duncan, G.J. & Newman, S. (1976). People as planners: The fulfillment of residential mobility expectations. In G.J. Duncan and J.N. Morgan (Eds.), *Five*

Thousand American Families–Patterns of Economic Progress, 3. Ann Arbor, MI: University of Michigan Institute for Social Research.

Easterlin, R.A., Macdonald, C., & Macunovich, D.J. (1990). Retirement prospects of the baby boom generation: A different perspective. *The Gerontologist, 30*(6), 776-783.

Eichner, M.M. & Morris, E.W. (1984). Energy conservation, air quality, health, and housing satisfaction. *Housing and Society, 11*(1), 1-15.

Erdner, R. & Guy, R. (1990). Career identification and women's attitudes toward retirement. *International Journal of Aging and Human Development, 30*(2), 129-139.

Fishbein, M. (Ed.). (1967). *In Attitude Theory and Measurement.* New York: John Wiley & Sons.

Gigy, L. (1986). Pre-retired and retired women's attitudes toward retirement. *International Journal of Aging and Human Development, 22*(1), 31-44.

Glazer, N. (1983). Housework. In L. Richardson and V. Taylor (Eds.), *Feminist Frontiers–Rethinking Sex, Gender, and Society.* Reading, MA: Addison-Wesley Publishing Co.

Goss, E.P., & Paul, C. (1986). Age and work experience in the decision to migrate. *The Journal of Human Resources, 21*(3), 399-405.

Grad, S. (1990, January). Income change at retirement. *Social Security* Bulletin, *53*(1).

Hurd, M.D. (1990). Research on the elderly: Economic status, retirement, and consumption and saving. *Journal of Economic Literature, 28,* 565-637.

Johnson-Carroll, K.J.A., Brandt, J.A., & Olson, G.I. (1987). Factors that influence energy-conservation alterations in Oregon households. *Housing and Society, 12*(2), 111-129.

Kart, C.S., Longino, C.F., & Ullmann, S.G. (1989). Comparing the economically advantaged and the pension elite: 1980 census profiles. *The Gerontologist, 29*(6), 745-749.

Kilty, K.J. & Behling, J. (1985). Predicting the retirement intentions and attitudes of professional workers. *Journal of Gerontology, 40*(2), 219-227.

Lee, E.S. (1980). Migration of the aged. *Research on Aging, 2*(2), 131-135.

Leonard-Barton, D. (1981). Voluntary simplicity lifestyles and energy. *Journal of Consumer Research, 8,* 243-252.

McFadden, J.R., Brandt, J.A., & Tripple, P.A. (1989). Housing for disabled persons: To what extent will today's homes accommodate a wheelchair? Paper presented at the American Association of Housing Educators Annual Conference, Greensboro, North Carolina.

Morris, E.W., & Jakubczak, M. (1988). Tenure-structure deficit, housing satisfaction and the propensity to move. *Journal of Marriage and the Family, 38,* 309-320.

Morris, E.W. and Winter, M. (1978). *Housing, family and society.* New York: John Wiley & Sons.

Morrison, B.M., Gladhart, P.M., Zuiches, J.H., Keith, J.G., Keefe, D. & Long,

B.R. (1978). Energy and families: The crisis and the response. *Journal of Home Economics, 70*, 19-21.

Patrick, C.H. (1980). Health and migration of the elderly. *Research on Aging, 2*(2), 233-241.

Pickvance, C.G. (1973). Life-cycle housing tenure and intra-urban residential mobility: A causal model. *The Sociological Review, 21*(2).

Prothero, J., & Beach, L.R. (1984). Retirement decisions: Expectation, intention, and action. *Journal of Applied Social Psychology, 14*(2), 162-174.

Reid, D.W., & Zeigler, M. (1980). Validity and stability of a new desired control measure pertaining to psychological adjustment to elderly. *Journal of Gerontology, 34*, 395-402.

Rhodes, S. (1983). Age related differences in work attitudes and behavior: A review and conceptual analysis. *Psychological Bulletin, 95*(2), 328-338.

Shaw, L. (1984). Retirement plans of middle-aged married women. *The Gerontologist, 24*(2), 301-313.

Szinovacz, M. (1986). Preferred retirement timing and retirement satisfaction in women. *International Journal of Aging and Human Development, 24*(4), 301-313.

Stern, P.C., Black, J.S., & Elworth, J.T. (1982, January). Influences on household energy adaptation: Investments, modifications, sacrifices. Paper presented in a symposium, Behavioral Approaches to Energy Conservation, at the meeting of the American Association for the Advancement of Science, Washington, D.C.

Tyler, L.L., Lovingood, R.P. Bowen, S.P. & Tyler, R.F. (1982). Energy-related characteristics of low-income urban tenants. *Housing and Society, 9*(3), 9-15.

Van Arsdol, M.D., Sabagh, G. & Butler, E.W. (1968). Retrospective and subsequent metropolitan residential mobility. *Demography, 5*, 249-267.

Walden, M.L. & Meeks, C.B. (1982). The demand for housing capital expenditures by the elderly. *Housing and Society, 9*, 31-41.

Wicker, A.W. (1969). Attitudes versus actions; The relationship of verbal and other behavioral responses to attitude objects. *Journal of Social Issues, 25*(4), 41-79.

Wilk, R.R. & Wilhite, H.L. (1983, October). Household energy decision-making in Santa Cruz County, California. In B.M. Morrison and W. Kempton (Eds.), *Proceedings of Families and Energy Coping with Uncertainty* (pp. 449-458). East Lansing, MI: Michigan State University.

Chapter 7

The Decision to Move to a Continuing Care Retirement Community

Nancy W. Sheehan
Rona J. Karasik

SUMMARY. The research examined factors related to the decision to move to a continuing care retirement community (CCRC). Employing a sample obtained from a recently opened comprehensive CCRC, 184 residents and 246 waiting list respondents were surveyed concerning their decision to move. Residents evidenced significantly more "risk" factors than waiting list applicants and reported significantly more reasons for selecting a CCRC. Reasons for choosing a CCRC were guaranteed health care, freedom from home maintenance, and supportive services. The vulnerability of residents requires careful attention for planning and managing services to maintain independence.

Nancy W. Sheehan, PhD, is Associate Professor, School of Family Studies, Travelers Center on Aging, University of Connecticut, Storrs, CT 06268. Rona J. Karasik, MA, is affiliated with the Department of Individual and Family Studies, University of Delaware, Newark, DE 19711.

An earlier version of this paper was presented at the 42nd Annual Meeting of the Gerontological Society of America, Minneapolis, MN, November, 17-21, 1989.

[Haworth co-indexing entry note]: "The Decision to Move to a Continuing Care Retirement Community." Sheehan, Nancy W., and Rona J. Karasik. Co-published simultaneously in *Journal of Housing for the Elderly* (The Haworth Press, Inc.) Vol. 11, No. 2, 1995, pp. 107-122; and: *Housing Decisions for the Elderly: To Move or Not to Move* (ed: Leon A. Pastalan) The Haworth Press, Inc., 1995, pp. 107-122. Multiple copies of this article/chapter may be purchased from The Haworth Document Delivery Center [1-800-3-HAWORTH; 9:00 a.m. - 5:00 p.m. (EST)].

Despite the rapid growth in the development of continuing care retirement communities (CCRCs), relatively little is known about the characteristics of CCRC residents and older persons' reasons for choosing a CCRC. CCRCs were developed to provide a planned housing alternative to meet the needs of older persons to maintain an independent lifestyle, while at the same time guaranteeing access to a range of long-term care services. A useful working definition of a CCRC is: ". . . a long-term alternative providing a package of services, including housing, health care and social services, to the elderly" (Schneider, 1987, p. 52). Four specific components are evident in CCRCs. These are: (1) the provision of independent living units; (2) a range of health care and social services which may include either intermediate or skilled nursing care; (3) some type of prepayment; and (4) a contract that describes the service obligations of the resident (Schneider, 1987; Winklevoss & Powell, 1984). As the concept of the CCRC residential alternative has emerged, three variations in service arrangements have evolved: (1) comprehensive; (2) modified; and (3) fee-for-service. Each type reflects differences in the availability of long-term services and the method of payment. The comprehensive model provides the full range of long-term services from independent living units to skilled nursing care. According to a recent industry report, comprehensive CCRCS or "all-inclusive contracts" account for one-third of all CCRCs (AAHA, 1981).

Estimates predict that the number of CCRCs will triple by the year 2000 (Schneider, 1987). Despite this rapid growth, there have been few research studies examining the psychosocial aspects of the decision to move to a CCRC or the adjustment of CCRC residents. Rather, the gerontological literature has primarily focused on either the financial solvency and long-term costs of CCRCs (Ruchlin, 1988) or legislative protection of the rights of older persons (Netting & Wilson, 1987). One recent study, however, did examine reasons for joining a CCRC. According to Cohen and his colleagues (1988), among persons joining a CCRC, the most important reason was "access to services that will help maintain my independence" (Cohen et al., 1988, p. 693). This study, however, failed to distinguish between reasons for joining a CCRC reported by recent residents and persons on the waiting list.

The present research, employing a sample of CCRC residents and waiting list respondents, is part of a longitudinal study examining factors related to adjustment to a CCRC. The specific questions addressed by the present investigation are: What differences exist between residents and persons on the waiting list for a CCRC? What are the reasons why older persons choose to move to a CCRC? What factors are involved in the decision-making process in deciding to move to a CCRC? Are there social and personality factors that are related to the decision to move?

METHODS

Sample

Respondents were 184 residents and 246 persons on the waiting list of a newly opened comprehensive CCRC. Both groups were predominantly female, 65% (residents) and 63.8% (waiting list). The average years of education for both groups were over 15 years of formal education (15.1 years, residents and 15.4 years, waiting list). Residents were significantly older than waiting list respondents ($t = 10.35$, $p < .0001$). The mean ages for residents and waiting list respondents were 79.7 and 73.4 years, respectively. Residents were also significantly less likely to be married (chi-square 13.4, $df = 4$, $p < .009$). In addition, residents' subjective health was significantly poorer than waiting list respondents' (chi-square 19.3, $df = 3$, $p < .000$). Table 1 presents a demographic profile of residents and applicants.

The majority of residents (88.6%) had moved to the CCRC from either their own home where they lived alone (37.9%) or the home they shared with their spouse (50.5%). Over 90% (93.8%) of CCRC applicants currently reside either in their home alone (30.7%) or with their spouse (63.1%). The majority of both residents (50.8%) and waiting list applicants (59.5%), respectively, reported that their previous or present home was located in the same city as the CCRC.

Comparison of the characteristics of the present sample to the profile of all residents in the facility and the AAHA's profile of CCRC residents indicates similarities and differences. While the average age of the sample, 79.7 years of age, matches the overall

TABLE 1. Demographic Profile of CCRC Residents and Applicants

	Resident	Waiting List
Age***	79.7 years	73.4 years
Gender		
female	65.5%	63.8%
male	34.5	36.2
Race		
White	100.0%	100.0%
Education	15.1 years	15.4 years
Marital status**		
married	50.3%	65.0%
widowed	37.2	26.4
divorced	2.7	4.1
ever-single	9.3	4.5
Religious Preference		
Catholic	29.5%	28.6%
Protestant	60.1	62.0
Jewish	2.7	3.3
Other	3.3	2.4
None	4.4	3.7
Subjective Health***		
poor	1.1%	–
fair	14.5	5.0
good	60.3	56.9
excellent	24.0	38.1

*** $p < .001$
** $p < .01$

age of the typical Northeast CCRC resident (79.8 years of age, AAHA, 1987), it is slightly younger than that of the total resident population for the CCRC (81.2, males and 80.3, females). The sex ratio of the present sample (65.5% female and 34.5% male) has a higher percentage of males than the AAHA figures from the Northeast region (75% and 25%) and a slightly higher percentage of males than the entire resident population (70% and 30%).

CCRC Research Site

The research site was a newly opened CCRC located in an affluent suburb of a metropolitan area in the Northeast. The facility provides independent units (N = 250) and guaranteed access to all levels of needed health care. At the time of the study, the entrance fee ranged from $68,000 for single occupancy of a studio unit to $142,000 for double occupancy of a two-bedroom unit. The accompanying monthly fee ranged from $1,125 to $2,230. Prior to the need for skilled nursing care, residents are provided health and support services in their own independent units. Skilled nursing care is provided in a nursing home located adjacent to the CCRC. Residents have priority access to this skilled nursing facility. If a nursing home bed is unavailable, reimbursement for skilled care at another facility will be provided.

Research Instruments

Two versions of a self-administered questionnaire (resident and waiting list) assessed demographic information (age, sex, marital status, living arrangements, religious preference); functional and subjective health status; availability of social support; housing satisfaction; persons and/or events that influenced the decision to move; reasons for moving; residential history (number of previous residential moves, length of time involved in the decision to move); service utilization; and locus of control beliefs (internal, chance and powerful others) (adapted from Sevenson, 1976). Individual subscales from the Multilevel Assessment Inventory assessed morale, social activity, and mobility (Lawton, n.d.).

PROCEDURE

The Resident Questionnaire was distributed to all residents three days after their move into the complex. Each resident was contacted by the Director of Nursing or one of her staff who explained the purpose of the study and distributed the questionnaire. Residents agreeing to participate signed an informed consent form. To ensure privacy, each resident was instructed to enclose the completed questionnaire in an attached envelope and place it sealed in a collection box located in a secure, central location.

Waiting list participants were contacted by mail. A cover letter explaining the purpose of the study and seeking cooperation and a stamped addressed envelope accompanied the questionnaire. All persons on the waiting list as of September 1988 were surveyed.

RESULTS

Differences Between Residents and Waiting List Respondents

As noted earlier, CCRC residents were older, in poorer health, experienced more functional limitations and were less likely to be married. Overall, the greater vulnerability of residents may be one of the major precipitating factors influencing the final decision to move to a CCRC.

Additional differences between the two groups support the finding of greater vulnerability of residents. Risk factors that significantly differentiated between residents and applicants were health, mobility, and availability of informal support. Residents were more likely to report that health problems interfered with their ability to do things they want to do (chi-square = 25.2, $df = 2$, p < .000). Over three times as many residents reported that health problems interfered "a great deal" with carrying out desired activities (12.8% vs. 2.9%). Residents (24.7%) were also more likely to report that their health had deteriorated during the past three years than waiting list respondents (13.7%) (chi-square = 8.19, $df = 2$, p < .017). Residents also reported greater limitations in their overall mobility (t = −2.16, p < .03).

Residents were less likely to have surviving adult children (chi-square = 3.64, $df = 1$, p < .06). There were no differences in emotional closeness, however, between resident and waiting list respondents with children. Residents reported having fewer family members available to provide help with shopping (t = −2.07, p < .04), advice (t = −2.43, p < .02), and financial management (t = −2.11, p < .04). Similarly, residents reported fewer friends to help when ill (t = −2.61, p < .01) or provide assistance with shopping (t = −2.94, p < .004).

There were no differences, however, in the number of family members to provide assistance when ill and the numbers of family or friends to provide emotional support. Overall, residents were significantly more likely than applicants to view the assistance that they receive from family as important (chi-square = 12.22, df = 2, p < .007).

REASONS FOR CHOOSING A CCRC

Reasons most frequently cited for choosing a CCRC were: guaranteed health care, freedom from home maintenance, supportive services, and personal safety/security. For both groups, the relative importance of reasons for choosing a CCRC is similar. Residents were significantly more likely to cite guaranteed health care as a major reason for their decision (chi-square = 6.13, df = 1, p < .01). Residents were somewhat more likely to report personal safety/security as a reason (chi-square = 3.66, df = 1, p < .056). Table 2 presents the frequency of reasons for deciding to move to a CCRC. Residents reported significantly more reasons for their decision to move to a CCRC (t = 3.49, p < .0005).

Separate analyses were conducted to examine the effects of age (under 75, 75 and over), marital status (married, unmarried), and

TABLE 2. Reasons for Decision to Move to a CCRC

Reason	Residents	Applicants
guaranteed health care*	95.6%	88.7%
freedom from home maintenance	82.8	80.2
supportive services	59.2	50.4
safety/security	47.8	38.3
independence from family	35.0	31.1
increased social opportunities	35.0	30.2
planned social activities	30.6	28.4
educational opportunities	28.3	26.1
convenient to family	23.9	26.1
loneliness	15.6	11.3

* x^2 = 6.13, (p < .01)

gender on the reasons for deciding to move to a CCRC (see Table 3). Age did not affect residents' reasons for deciding to move. Age, however, was significantly related to applicants' reasons for selecting a CCRC. Younger persons on the waiting list were more likely to cite independence from family, increased opportunities for social interaction, and educational opportunities as reasons for moving to a CCRC. Older waiting list respondents were more likely to cite planned social activities.

Marital status affected reasons for choosing a CCRC. Unmarried resident and waiting list respondents were more likely to cite safety/security, increased opportunities for social opportunities, planned social activities, and loneliness, while married residents were more likely to cite guaranteed health care.

Gender also affected reasons for deciding to move to a CCRC, particularly for the waiting list respondents. Women on the waiting list were more likely to mention: safety/security, independence from family, increased social opportunities, educational opportunities, convenience to family, and loneliness. For residents, women were more likely than men to cite safety/security and independence from family as reasons for their decision.

DECISION-MAKING REGARDING THE MOVE TO A CCRC

In order to explore the decision-making process concerning moving to a CCRC, the present study examined respondents' perceived difficulty in making the decision, whether persons or events had influenced their decision, concerns about moving to a CCRC, and whether individual differences in locus of control were related to aspects of the decision-making process.

As the number of reasons attributed to the decision to move increased, the difficulty involved in making the decision decreased ($r = -.21$, $p < .0001$). Respondents who reported more reasons were more likely to report that a person/event influenced their decision ($r = .14$, $p < .008$). Those who reported more reasons had also been thinking about the possibility of moving from their home for a longer time ($r = .16$, $p < .002$) and viewed family assistance as more important ($r = .13$, $p < .01$).

TABLE 3. Resident and Waiting List Respondents' Reasons for Deciding to Move to a CCRC by Age, Marital Status and Gender

	Resident		Waiting List	
AGE	under 75	75+ older	under 75	75+ older
guaranteed health care	96.7%	95.7%	92.0%	83.7%
freedom from home maintenance	90.0	80.8	82.1	78.6
supportive services	73.3	55.7	45.5	56.1
safety/security	56.7	46.1	35.7	43.9
independence from family	46.7	34.0	37.5	24.5*
increased social opportunities	36.7	36.2	22.3	41.8**
planned social activities	26.7	31.9	20.5	38.8**
education opportunities	40.0	24.8	33.0	17.3**
convenient to family	26.7	24.1	26.8	25.5
loneliness	20.0	15.6	9.8	13.3

MARITAL STATUS	Married	Unmarried	Married	Unmarried
guaranteed health care	98.9	92.1*	90.3	85.9
freedom from home maintenance	84.4	80.9	82.6	75.6
supportive services	60.0	57.9	48.6	53.8
safety/security	38.9	57.3**	31.2	51.3**
independence from family	37.8	32.6	29.9	33.3
increased social opportunities	20.0	50.6****	25.0	39.7*
planned social activities	21.1	40.4**	24.3	35.9
education opportunities	27.8	29.2	21.5	34.6*
convenient to family	26.7	21.3	25.7	26.9
loneliness	1.1	30.3****	4.2	24.4****

TABLE 3 (continued)

GENDER	Resident		Waiting List	
	Male	Female	Male	Female
guaranteed health care	94.9	95.5	86.4	90.1
freedom from home maintenance	83.0	82.1	81.5	79.4
supportive services	57.6	59.5	42.0	55.3
safety/security	35.6	52.7*	25.9	45.4**
independence from family	25.4	41.1*	22.2	36.2*
increased social opportunities	25.4	39.3	18.5	36.9**
planned social activities	27.1	33.0	16.0	35.5
education opportunity	20.3	33.0	13.6	33.3***
convenient to family	16.9	28.6	18.5	30.5*
loneliness	10.2	17.0	3.7	15.6**

****p < .000
***p < .001
**p < .01
*p < .05

Since residents and applicants occupy different positions relative to the actual move, separate analyses were performed for each group to determine factors related to the decision. Waiting list respondents reported significantly greater difficulty in making the decision to move (chi-square = 17.68, $df = 2$, $p < .000$). Fourteen percent of the residents compared to approximately one-quarter of the waiting list respondents (24.2%) reported their decision was "very difficult." Residents who reported more reasons for joining experienced less difficulty in making their decision ($r = -.15$, $p < .05$) and had been thinking about moving for a longer time ($r = .19$, $p < .01$). Residents' greater satisfaction with their previous housing was related to attributing fewer reasons for their decision ($r = -.19$, $p < .01$). Satisfaction, however, was not related to the difficulty of the decision. Housing satisfaction was related to residents' morale ($r = .22$, $p < .004$), health ($r = .23$, $p < .002$), social activity ($r = .17$, $p < .03$) and mobility ($r = .16$, $p < .03$).

For waiting list respondents, more reported reasons for joining a CCRC was related to less difficulty of the decision in making the decision (r = −.23, p < .001) and the likelihood that the decision had been influenced by either a particular person/event (r = .25, p < .0005). Overall satisfaction with present housing was unrelated to either difficulty involved in making the decision to move or number of reasons cited for the decision to move. Variables correlated with waiting list respondents' housing satisfaction were age (r = −.17, p < .009), education (r = .18, p < .001), morale (r = .20, p < .002), health (r = .16, p < .01), social activity (r = .20, p < .001), and mobility (r = .23, p < .0001).

Over half of the combined sample (55.5%) reported that either an event or person had influenced their decision. Similar percentages of residents and applicants reported that their decision to join had been influenced by an event/person (53.7% and 56.8%, respectively). Table 4 presents the persons or events that influenced the decision to move. Residents were twice as likely to report that a change in their health had influenced the decision (25.5% vs. 10%) (chi-square = 9.32, df = 1, p < .002). Residents were also more likely to mention either changes in spouse's health (16.7% vs. 8.3%, chi-square = 3.58, df = 1, p < .06) and loneliness (15.7% vs. 8.3%, chi-square = 2.88, df = 1, p < .09) as events influencing their decision. Overall, the most frequently cited influence was a friend, 26.7% and 34.2%, of residents and applicants, respectively. Family members, children and spouse, were more frequently mentioned by residents as influencing their decision. More specifically, children were mentioned by 23.8% of residents and 15.8% of waiting list respondents, while a spouse was mentioned by 23.8% and 18.3% of resident and waiting list respondents, respectively.

Based upon responses to an open-ended question, residents were more likely to express concerns about their overall adjustment or happiness living in a CCRC (chi-square = 17.97, df = 1, p < .000), ability to get around/health (chi-square = 16.87, df = 1, p < .000), and lack of outdoor space (chi-square = 4.02, df = 1, p < .04). Waiting list respondents were more likely to express concerns focused on the lack of space in individual units (chi-square = 31.8, df = 1, p < .000) and the age-segregated environment (chi-square = 8.05, df = 1, p < .005) (Table 5).

TABLE 4. Persons or Events Reported as Influencing the Decision to Move to a CCRC

	Residents	Waiting List
Person		
friend	26.7%	34.2%
spouse	23.8	18.3
child	23.8	15.8
other relative	4.9	8.3
Event		
change in health	25.5	10.0**
death of spouse	17.5	17.5
spouse's health	16.7	8.3*
loneliness	15.7	8.3

**p < .002
*p < .06

LOCUS OF CONTROL
AND THE DECISION-MAKING PROCESS

Overall, the specific pattern of interrelationships among control beliefs and factors related to the decision-making process indicated people with a strong internal locus of control were more likely to be satisfied with their housing ($r = .13$, $p < .01$) and less likely to indicate that they had been influenced by a person/event in making their decision ($r = -.19$, $p < .0009$). While persons who believe that what happens is influenced by chance were less satisfied with their housing ($r = -.13$, $p < .006$) and reported more reasons for their decision to move ($r = .20$, $p < .0001$). Finally, a belief in powerful others was generally unrelated to decision-making factors. Only housing satisfaction was related to a belief in powerful others ($r = -.16$, $p < .002$).

Separate correlations examining the relationship between control beliefs and decision-making were performed for the resident and waiting list groups. For residents, internality was related to the likelihood of not being influenced by events/persons in their decision making process ($r = -.26$, $p < .003$). Age was positively related to an internal belief system ($r = .16$, $p < .05$). The belief in chance was related to lowered satisfaction with previous housing ($r = -.34$, $p < .0001$) and poorer subjective health ($r = -.20$, $p < .006$). Finally, a belief in powerful others was also related to lower hous-

TABLE 5. Concerns Expressed About Moving to a CCRC

	Residents	Waiting List
adjustment	41.8%	22.8%***
health	24.5	9.8***
privacy	10.9	15.0
financial	10.3	14.6
interior space	7.1	28.9***
outdoor space	4.9	10.2*
quality of care	7.1	7.3
food	4.9	4.5
age-segregated environment	1.6	7.7**

*** p < .000
**p < .005
*p < .05

ing satisfaction (r = − .27, p < .0005). Powerful others was also related to age (r = .24, p < .002), morale (r = − .15, p < .05), and health (r = − .17, p < .03).

For the waiting list group, an internal belief system was related to greater difficulty in making the decision (r = .21, p < .005) and greater overall housing satisfaction (r = .14, p < .04). Other factors related to greater internality were sex (r = .14, p < .03) and morale (r = .20, p < .004). A belief in chance was related to increased reasons cited for the move to a CCRC. Mobility was also related to chance (r = .21, p < .0009). Powerful others was unrelated to any of the housing decision-making variables. A belief in powerful others was related to age (r = .16, p < .02), morale (r = − .24, p < .0004) and health (r = − .15, p < .03).

DISCUSSION

The results of the present study suggest that complex processes underlie the decision to move to a CCRC. While CCRC residents possess significantly more risk factors (poorer health, single marital status, older, limited mobility, and fewer informal supports), resident and waiting list respondents identified similar reasons for the decision to move to a CCRC. However, residents reported more reasons for their decision and had been thinking about moving for a considerably longer period of time. For persons who decide to live in a CCRC, the decision to leave their home appears to be made over a long period of time. Among CCRC residents, marital status and gender, but not age, influenced their reasons for choosing a CCRC. More specifically, unmarried residents more frequently cited socially-related reasons (loneliness, planned social activities, and social opportunities), safety, and health care than married residents as reasons for their move, while female residents were more likely to mention safety and independence from family.

Among waiting list residents, gender had the most widespread influence. Female applicants to a CCRC were more likely than men to cite safety, social opportunities, independence from family, educational opportunities, convenience to family, and loneliness as reasons for their decision. Unmarried applicants, in comparison to their married peers, more frequently cited safety, social opportunities, loneliness, and educational opportunities. Finally, older applicants placed greater value on planned social activities and social opportunities, while younger applicants cited educational opportunities and independence from family. Obviously, the salient reasons for moving to a CCRC vary among older persons. Of all factors, marital status had the most pervasive influence.

Thus, for persons moving to a CCRC, the decision-making process appears to extend over a long period of time and involves differential perceptions of the advantages of living in a CCRC. The move to a CCRC may be precipitated by increased frailty, decreased mobility, limited informal support, and a desire not to be dependent on adult children. The long-term process of deciding to move to a CCRC holds strong implications for the viabilility of the CCRC system which depends upon the majority of its tenants at any given time being healthy and making relatively few demands upon the CCRC's health care services. If potential residents tend to significantly delay their move to the CCRC, they are likely to be older, less healthy, and require more health services upon arrival. Such an incoming population would undoubtedly place a strain on the

CCRCs' financial projections for supporting its tenants. Given the cross-sectional nature of the comparison, we can only speculate whether certain risk factors may precipitate the decision for older persons to move to a CCRC. An 18-month follow-up of waiting list applicants which is currently underway will help to identify the significant factors associated with the decision-making process. Clearly, the decision to move is not a straightforward one. The rapid growth in the development of CCRCs, however, indicates that developers feel that the decision to move to a CCRC will be an increasingly popular one among affluent older persons.

The most common concerns expressed by respondents in the present investigation concerning the move to a CCRC (adjustment to the facility, maintenance of health, and privacy) did not resemble the major concerns identified by previous researchers. According to Cohen et al. (1988), the most frequent concerns about joining a CCRC were financial in nature (ability to keep up with the entrance fee, the size of the entrance fee, and size of the monthly fee). Based upon the findings of the present study, different concerns expressed by residents and applicants reflect their different position relative to the actual move to a CCRC.

Finally, consideration must also be given to the unusual composition of the CCRC population. As suggested by the financial requirements of CCRC living, and supported by the findings of the present study, CCRC tenants and potential (waiting list) tenants tend to have higher educational and socioeconomic statuses than the general elderly population. As a group, so-called affluent elders are not often studied by gerontologists, making comparisons and generalizations from CCRC studies to studies of other types of senior housing somewhat limited. Further study of both CCRCs and high status elderly is warranted.

REFERENCES

American Association of Homes for the Aging and Ernst and Whinney. (1987). Continuing care retirement communities: An industry in action. Analysis and developing trends. Washington, DC: Scott Foresman and Company, Glenview, IL.

Cohen, M., Tell, E., Batten, H. & Larson, M. (1988). Attitudes toward joining continuing care retirement communities. *The Gerontologist, 28*, 637-643.

Lawton, M. P. (n.d.). Multidimensional Assessment Inventory. Philadelphia: Philadelphia Geriatric Center.

Levenson, H. (1976). Activism and powerful others: Distinctions within the concept of internal-external control. *Journal of Personality Assessment, 38,* 377-383.

Netting, F. E. & Wilson, E. (1987). Current legislation concerning life care and continuing care contracts. *The Gerontologist, 27,* 645-651.

Ruchlin, H. (1988). Continuing care retirement communities: An analysis of financial viability and health care coverage. *The Gerontologist, 28,* 156-162.

Schneider, R. (1987). Financial and management factors affecting CCRCs long-term viability. *Contemporary Long-Term Care, 10,* 52-58.

Winklevoss, W. & Powell, A. (1984). *Continuing care retirement communities:* An empirical, financial, and legal analysis. Homewood, IL: Richard D. Irwin.

Chapter 8

Home Builders' Attitudes and Knowledge of Aging: The Relationship to Design for Independent Living

Suzanne H. Belser
Joseph A. Weber

SUMMARY. This study examined the relationship between home builders' attitudes/knowledge of aging and their awareness/use of accessible products and features in residential design. Eighty-nine Oklahoma home builders completed a comprehensive survey that included demographics, building practices, and Palmore's FAQII. The mean score for knowledge of aging was 12.5 out of 25. The net-bias mean score for attitude showed a tendency for the sample to think negatively about the elderly. A conceptual model to predict use and knowledge was developed and tested using multiple regression analysis. Results indicated that home builders were aware of a higher percentage of accessible features than they actually used. The majority of builders reported that accessible features in a residence was a viable idea but their use depended on client awareness and request.

Suzanne H. Belser is Graduate Research Assistant and Dr. Joseph A. Weber is Associate Professor, both with the Department of Family Relation and Child Development, College of Human Environmental Services, Oklahoma State University, Stillwater, OK 74078-0337.

[Haworth co-indexing entry note]: "Home Builders' Attitudes and Knowledge of Aging: The Relationship to Design for Independent Living." Belser, Suzanne H., and Joseph A. Weber. Co-published simultaneously in *Journal of Housing for the Elderly* (The Haworth Press, Inc.) Vol. 11, No. 2, 1995, pp. 123-137; and: *Housing Decisions for the Elderly: To Move or Not to Move* (ed: Leon A. Pastalan) The Haworth Press, Inc., 1995, pp. 123-137. Multiple copies of this article/chapter may be purchased from The Haworth Document Delivery Center [1-800-3-HAWORTH; 9:00 a.m. - 5:00 p.m. (EST)].

The increase in the proportion of older people has generated concern about their ability to function and live independently. In the near future, traditional forms of institutional care, such as nursing homes, boarding houses and psychiatric hospitals will not be viable solutions to long term care due to the vast population of elderly people (Null, 1989).

Developmental and physiological changes that occur with age have an impact on the ability of older people to function in the community and carry out activities of daily living (Czaja, 1988). The environment in which one lives can aid or hinder these basic activities such as dressing, bathing and eating. Researchers have recognized that design of the physical environment plays a major role in the ability of an elderly person to continue to perform daily tasks and thereby to continue to live independently (Andreasen, 1985; Lawton, 1989). The ability to carry out daily activities is a major factor in a family's or health professional's assessment of an older person's ability to function independently. Results from such assessments play a role in recommending continued independence versus institutionalization (Altman, Lawton & Wohlwill, 1984).

Institutionalization is costly in human and economic terms. In human terms, the majority of elderly people value their independence and prefer to age in their own homes (Shapiro & Tate, 1988). "Aging in place" allows people to continue to enjoy privacy, independence and be in control of their lives and maintain the comfort and familiarity of the home and neighborhood in which they live. It has been documented that the environment in which people live can contribute to their emotional health and well being (Andreasen, 1985; Lawton, 1989). This is especially true for home environments of the elderly because the amount of discretionary time spent inside the home increases with age; up to 80-90% of their time each day is spent in their homes (AARP, 1990b, 1992; Czaja, 1988).

In terms of economics, as the proportion of the elderly population increases, the problem of institutionalization and its cost may assume even greater importance (Kahana, 1974). The national average for skilled and intermediate nursing home care ranges from $1,400 to $2,000 per month (National Center for Health Statistics, [NCHS], 1991). Therefore, aging at home will become an increasingly viable solution. Families, as well as builders and other housing professionals, would benefit from understanding the advantages of home designs that allow individuals to remain living independently for the maximum period of time. Residential environments that are accessible and functional for all people without regard to age, ability or physical limitations can aid in life-long tenancy. By routinely incorporating universal design features which are supportive, adaptable, accessible, and provide for life safety, a total life-span environment can be economically achieved (Beitz, Kirby, & Brewer, 1992).

The purpose of this study is to provide a better understanding of the factors that affect current design and construction practices, which do not typically facilitate life-long use, of single family homes. Specific objectives include:

1. to determine the builders' level of knowledge and attitude of aging and whether they have an effect on the awareness or use of accessible features in residential design;
2. to determine the builders' awareness level and use of accessible products and features and how these correlate with each other.

REVIEW OF RELEVANT LITERATURE

Housing and Independence

Planned housing and institutions constitute only a small portion of where older people live. Today the proportion of elderly people living in institutions is around five percent. Remaining in place is by far the most frequent choice made by older people when making decisions about where to live. However, past and current building practices do not promote the concept of "aging in place." There is a growing concern of how older people will deal with their existing housing in ordinary neighborhoods (Lawton & Hoover, 1981; Struyk, 1977). The development of a new approach to housing must begin with an understanding of what it means to grow old in our society.

Health and Independent Living

The life cycle is a process of biological, psychological and social change which requires constant adaption by individuals and the environments in which they live (Hoglund, 1983; Lawton, 1989). The change occurs at different rates for different people, which makes chronological age a poor indicator of physical age and change (Salmon, 1963; Gunn, 1988; Ferrini & Ferrini, 1989). There are individuals in all age groups who experience some disability or impairment. For most of the population, the aging process does lead to a gradual decline in functioning and an increase in dependence, due to changes in vision, hearing, mobility, agility, strength, endurance and dexterity. However, increased dependence does not necessarily mean a loss of independence (Hoglund, 1983). Physical environments can be designed or modified to accommodate these changes (Hartford Insurance Group, [HIG], 1990). The built environment can help maximize the control older people have over their surroundings and reduce their sense of helplessness (Christenson, 1990). Losing their independence due to health reasons is a fear that many older adults have. Independence and the ability to control one's environment have been found to be powerful variables in human behavior. Enhanced control has been related to enhanced self-esteem. Identifying ways to maintain control is essential to the well being of the elderly (Barques, Waxman, & Yaffe, 1988).

The Meaning of Home

The home has special significance for older persons; it is a meaningful expression of their personal and social self and holds much emotional significance (Michelson, 1977; Cooper-Marcus, 1974; Dangelis & Fengler, 1990). Researchers have observed that an older person's home represents a reservoir of family history and memorabilia (Csikszentmihalyi & Rochberg-Halton, 1981). Remaining in the family home perpetuates a sense of tradition and preserves self-esteem (O'Bryant, 1983). To be forced to leave this familiar and secure environment means losing memories, independence and control.

Secure environments may be tied to economic issues. Of the ninety-five percent of American elders who live in non-institutional settings, seventy-five percent own the dwelling in which they live (AARP, 1990b; Callahan, 1992). Since most elderly home owners have paid off their mortgage, the home is also a great economic asset (Danigelis & Fengler, 1990). In a recent AARP survey of consumer preferences, concerns and needs, a significant finding was that the preference for aging-in-place is prevalent among older people. Eighty-six percent said they wanted to stay in their present home and never move (AARP, 1990b).

Gerontologists have shown particular interest in how much the elderly's morale or life satisfaction is influenced by their residential environment. Residential well being is closely related to psychological well being (Lawton, 1989). Research has shown that the elderly spend eighty to ninety percent of their day at home (AARP, 1990b; Gabb, Lodel, & Combs, 1991). The home environment is a physical setting for life's events, and plays a major part in an individual's hopes and dreams (Hoglund, 1983).

Current Practices

Traditionally, individuals have had to adapt in order to "fit" an environment, instead of adapting the environment to "fit" the individual (Null, 1989; Brent & Brent, 1987). Most older people live in standard, conventionally built, single-family detached dwellings that were built prior to 1950 (AARP, 1990a). The market for these houses is generally targeted at people in the 30-55 year old age range. This housing type has been described as "Peter Pan" housing. The name conveys the concept that the housing was designed for people who will never grow old (Hare, 1992). Living spaces have long been designed for use by one "average" physical type, the young, fit, adult male (Pastalan, 1988). The majority of standards and design practices in use prior to the 1950's have continued into the 1990's and do not respond to the needs and requirements of a large segment of the population. This is true not only for standard "spec" housing but also for custom built homes. Research indicates that the elderly make very few alterations to their living environments; therefore they may live in places not suitable for their needs (Beitz, Kirby & Brewer, 1992; Brent, Lower-Walker, & Twaddell, 1983).

Historically, home builders have not seen the environment as part of a support system in assessing or responding to an individual's needs, and seldom recommend that changes in standards be made (Hiatt, 1984). Instead, builders focus on the tangible features of a home, such as the structure and the visual aesthetics. They have very little concern about interaction between the environment and the person (Hoglund, 1983).

Although most home builders seem to understand that the environment has an effect on the user, few give this much consideration when designing (Gabb et al., 1991). In a study by Reizenstein (1975), most of the designers surveyed were aware of environment and behavior research and believed that the environment influences behavior. However, few of the designers had ever used the research findings in their work. They did not incorporate the findings because the findings were not readily available or were written in "jargon-like" language, and the implications for design were not immediately obvious.

Sommer (1974) identifies several explanations for the reluctance of professionals to pay attention to the values and needs of the occupants. He suggests that rather than trying to accommodate the varied needs of different types of users, it is easier for builders to assume that everyone has similar needs and tastes. Home builders are often supplier oriented and are most interested in persuading users to accept the designs they want to supply (Gabb et al., 1991). For all individuals, habits and values are slow to change; there is no exception concerning the use of conventional building practices. Many home builders build according to building paradigms that are based on tradition. Builders are often unwilling to part from tradition long enough to see alternative ways of doing things.

Alternative Practice

The concept of universal design is based on the idea that design can meet the needs of all people, regardless of age, allowing them to achieve some balance of dependence and independence despite permanent or temporary disabilities (Null, 1989; McLeister, 1989; Hoglund, 1983; Mace, Hardie, & Place, 1990). During the course of their lives most people will need, at least temporarily, a supportive environment similar to that needed by the elderly (Gunn, 1988). Universal design features fit these needs since they offer support, they are adaptable, accessible and they provide life safety (Raschko, 1987). Examples of universal design features include, but are not limited to, the following: package shelves at entries, level thresholds, wide door openings, wide hallways, lever handled faucets and door hardware, ground level entry, low pile carpet, non-skid floors, adjustable counter heights, anti-scald devices, reinforced walls for grab bars, and shower or tub with built-in seating. Universal design has received support and its use in construction promoted and encouraged by the United States Department of Housing and Urban Development (HUD) and The American Society of Interior Designers (ASID) (HUD, 1988).

The Fair Housing Act of 1988 incorporates the principles of universal design. However, the law only applies to residential buildings containing over four units. Smaller buildings and single family homes are exempt from the law (Pynoos, 1992). Demographic trends in the United States today will increase the need for single family housing that will meet the needs of people of all ages and various disabilities (Gunn, 1988; Lueck, 1987).

The Consumer Market

Over half (53%) of older Americans have done little or no planning for their housing needs in later years (AARP, 1990b). There is a reluctance on the part of consumers to admit to the possibility of their needs changing as they age. To make an informed decision about future housing, an individual needs an understanding of the physical and emotional changes that occur with age. Consumers need to be aware of how the environment interacts with their needs and should learn to evaluate a design in terms of its effect on their needs as they grow older (Gabb et al., 1991). If the consumers could communicate their preferences more effectively, home builders might find it more profitable to accommodate them (Gunn, 1988).

Until recently there has not been a large number of elderly-specific or universal design products available. However, recent data from census reports, indicating the increasing population size and purchasing power of the elderly, have stimulated new interest in investments related to older people (Hiatt, 1988a). Today there are a wide variety of products on the market that assist in independent living but few are actually used in construction.

METHODOLOGY

This study was designed to determine if a home builder's knowledge and attitudes of aging, and awareness of products and features affect the design of single family homes. The findings of this study give a better understanding of the reasons why accessibility in private residences is not a standard practice in the building industry. Although the problem of providing housing that promotes independence for aging adults, as well as for young children and the disabled, is not new, little is known about why standard housing has not changed to accommodate their needs.

The Sample

The sample for this survey was obtained from the membership list of the Oklahoma Home Builders Association (OHBA). From the total membership list of 2000 which included realtors, commercial and residential builders, as well as contractors and architects, 200 members were randomly selected. One hundred surveys (50% of the target population) were returned to the researcher; of these, eleven surveys had incomplete data and could not be used. Eighty-nine surveys were analyzed in this survey.

The majority of the sample were males ranging in age from thirty to over fifty years (see Table 1). Most were college graduates, and reported their professional title as general contractors who had been in practice from eleven to twenty years. A majority of their work was residential and they built mainly custom homes ranging in size from 1000 s.f. to over 3000 s.f.

Instrumentation

The survey was divided into three sections; Background Information (demographics), Palmore's Facts on Aging Quiz II, and Design Awareness and Use. The first section of the survey included demographic information. This section also included typical construction costs and percentage of construction that was residential.

The second section of the survey used the Palmore Facts on Aging Quiz II (Palmore, 1977). The FAQ II scales were made up of

TABLE 1. Demographic Characteristics of Home Builders

Characteristics	Number	Percentages
Gender		
female	7	8.1
male	79	91.9
Age		
under 30	3	3.4
31-40	29	33.0
41-50	28	31.8
51-60	19	21.6
over 60	9	10.2
Education		
High school graduate	10	11.2
Some college	25	28.1
College graduate	41	31.8
Graduate or professional degree	12	21.6
Other	1	10.2
Tenure (years in practice)		
0-10	19	21.3
11-20	44	49.4
21-30	19	21.3
over 30	7	7.9
Title		
General contractor	76	85.4
Other (architect, sub-contractor)	13	14.6
Percentage of Residential Work		
0-25%	4	4.5
26-50%	6	6.8
51-75%	12	13.6
75-100%	66	75.0
Category of Residential Work		
Spec	19	21.3
Custom	66	74.2
Other	4	4.5
Client Age Range		
20-30	1	1.1
31-40	36	40.9
41-50	43	48.9
over 50	8	9.1

factual statements that can be documented by empirical research. The scales were designed to cover basic physical, mental, and social facts in addition to common misconceptions about aging. The FAQ II is composed of 25 fixed choice questions, which have true/false, and don't know responses. The survey was used to measure and compare levels of knowledge and misconceptions about aging. The FAQ II also served as an indirect measure of attitude towards the aged. The third section of the instrument, developed by the researcher, consisted of a total of 36 questions pertaining to the awareness and use of universal design-based products and features that enhance independent living.

FINDINGS

Knowledge of Aging

The mean knowledge score (Table 2) on the FAQII was 12.51 out of a possible 25. The scores ranged from a low of 2 to a high of 18. The mean attitude score (percentage of positive errors minus the percentage of negative errors) was -24.97. This net-bias score indicates that the sample of builders tend to think negatively about the elderly. Out of a potential high score of 108, the mean score on the awareness section was 61.74 and the mean score for the use section was 74.33.

Multiple regression analysis was performed involving the criterion variable awareness and the predictor variables knowledge, attitude, and the demographic variables: gender, age, years in practice, education, and occupation. One variable, attitude (net-bias), was found to be approaching significance at the .15 level ($p = .1239$, F = 2.42). The model explained 3.5% of the variance ($R^2 = .0305$). The builders who had a more negative attitude of aging tended to be less aware of accessible products and features.

Pearson's correlation coefficient was used to determine the association between selected variables. Age was found to have a significant positive relationship with years in practice ($p < .01$), and attitude ($p < .01$). Those respondents who were older tended to have been in the construction business longer and have a less positive attitude of aging. Awareness was found to be significantly related to years in practice ($p < .02$), and use ($p < .01$). Those respondents

TABLE 2. Mean Responses to the Facts on Aging Quiz II

Statement Content	Response Percent		
	True	False	Don't know
1 height declines	91	7	2
2 chronic illness	92	7	1
3 acute illness	46	36	18
4 injuries	64	27	9
5 absenteeism	6	80	14
6 black life expectancy	10	72	18
7 men's life expectancy	2	93	5
8 medicare	55	21	24
9 social security benefits	43	48	9
10 supplemental security benefits	31	40	29
11 share of nation's income	38	44	18
12 victimization	72	18	10
13 fear of crime	89	1	10
14 law abiding	89	3	8
15 number of widows/widowers	6	83	11
16 voting	70	18	12
17 public office	36	42	22
18 proportion of blacks	63	17	20
19 decline in participation	15	73	12
20 life alone	39	45	16
21 general poverty rate	19	64	17
22 black poverty rate	67	8	25
23 reduced activity	1	93	6
24 adjustment to empty nest	56	33	11
25 proportion widowed	31	45	24

	Mean	Standard Deviation
FAQII-Knowledge	12.516	3.506
FAQII-Attitude (Net-bias)	− 24.97	19.311

Note: Underlined values represent correct answer for that statement.

who had worked in the building industry the longest tended to be less aware of products and features. Respondents that reported more awareness correspondingly reported a higher incidence of use of features and products.

IMPLICATIONS

Historically, society has underestimated the need for housing that encourages independent living. Society has been too protective and has promoted helplessness rather than independence (Gunn, 1988). This phenomenon can be seen in the reluctance of the building industry to design houses that promote independence and may defer institutionalization. In order to change the current industry standards, home builders need to understand their present building paradigms and move on to new ones based on real needs rather than tradition.

The findings of this study supported the idea of the reluctance of builders to break from traditional building practices. Those respondents who had worked in the building industry the longest tended to be less aware of accessible products and features. In addition, those respondents who were older tended to have been in the construction business longer and had a more negative attitude of aging. These findings suggest that the home building industry would benefit in actively pursuing builders for educational programs concerning aging and accessibility. Although information is now available to builders, few seek it.

Two other variables that appear to be related to use of accessible features, are consumer demand and cost. Since consumer demand depends largely on knowledge, educational materials should be made easily available to the consumer when deciding to build a house. The home building industry, specifically home builders such as architects and contractors who deal with and influence clients, should have this material available to give to potential clients. The builder should stress the importance and conveniences of accessible designs and future needs should be discussed with the client.

It is hoped that accessible features will become standard items in residential environments. As these items are used more frequently and appreciated, the cost increase will become less of a deterrent.

Realistic and continually updated cost assessments for accessible features should also be outlined for different regions of the country and made available to builders and consumers.

With the recent passage of the American Disabilities Act much attention has been given to accessible environments for public spaces. It seems that the timing is right for the home building industry to take this one step further and apply accessible design techniques to the private housing industry. In the future, there should be some form of design regulations imposed on the building of single-family residences, just as there is for public spaces. Expanding the Fair Housing Act to cover single family homes would be a positive step toward a nationwide movement to promote universally designed housing. Many problems that existing homes present for "aging in place" would be eliminated if supportive, adaptable and accessible housing were built to begin with.

Incentives from the Federal government might spur home builders to use accessible features in construction of single family homes. Tax breaks for consumers may heighten the awareness and demand for these features, much in the same way as energy efficiency and fire safety were introduced to consumers. Insurance companies could play a major role in the promotion of the use of accessible features by reducing rates for owners of safe and accessible designed houses.

The demographic trends of an aging population will increase the need for new long term housing options. Independent living will no doubt be an option that many will choose. The home building industry in the United States must come to recognize and deal with the special needs of the aging population.

REFERENCES

Altman, I., Lawton, P. M. & Wohlwill, J. (Eds.) (1984). *Elderly people and the environment: Human behavior and development: advances in theory and research.* New York, NY: Plenum Press.

American Association of Retired Persons. (1992). *A profile of older Americans.* Washington, DC: Program Resources Department, AARP.

American Association of Retired Persons. (1990). *Your choice, your home: A workbook for older people and their families.* Washington, DC: American Association of Retired Persons Fulfillment Publications.

American Association of Retired Persons. (1990). *Understanding senior housing.* Washington, DC: Consumer Affairs Section Program Department Publication.

Andreasen, M. E. (1985). Make a safe environment by design. *Journal of Gerontological Nursing, 11*(6), 18-22.

Barques, M. A., Waxman, R. & Yaffe, L. (1988). The effects of a resident self-help model on control, social involvement and self-esteem among the elderly. *The Gerontologist, 28*, 620-624.

Beitz, B., Kirby, S., & Brewer, G. (1992). *Universal design: Acceptance of housing providers and housing consumers.* (Unpublished manuscript, Oklahoma State University.)

Brent, E., & Brent, R. (1987). ERHAP: An artificial intelligence expert system for assessing the housing of elderly residents. *Housing and Society, 14*(3), 215-230.

Brent, R. S., Lower-Walker, D. & Twaddell, N. (1983). Environmental adequacy and environmental adaptions. *Housing and Society, 10*(3), 135-140.

Callahan, J. (1992). Aging in Place. *Generations,* Spring, 5-6.

Center for Accessible Housing (1993). *The universal home series: Homes for living, homes for life.* Raleigh, NC: NCSU School of Design.

Cooper-Marcus, C. (1974). The house as a symbol of self. In Jon Lang, C. Burnette, W. Moleski, and D. Vachon (Eds.), *Designing for human behavior: Architecture and the behavioral sciences* (pp. 130-146). Stroudsburg, PA: Dowden, Hutchinson & Ross.

Christenson, M. (1990). Adaption of the physical environment to compensate for sensory changes. *Aging and the designed environment.* New York: The Haworth Press, Inc.

Csikszentmihalyi, M., & Rochberg-Halton, E. (1981). *The meaning of things.* New York: Cambridge University Press.

Czaja, S. (1988). Safety and security of the elderly: Implications for smart house design. *International Journal of Technology and Aging, 1*(1), 49-67.

Danigelis, N., & Fengler, A. (1990). Homesharing: How social exchange helps elders live at home. *The Gerontologist, 30*, 162-170.

Ferrini, A. F., & Ferrini, R. L. (1989). *Health in the later years.* Dubuque, IA: William C. Brown Publishers.

Gabb, B., Lodel, K. A., & Combs, E. R. (1991). User input in housing design: The interdisciplinary challenge. *Home Economics Research Journal, 20*, 16-25.

Gunn, B. (1988). Housing for an aging society: How relevant is age? *Housing and Society, 15*(3), 246-253.

Hare, P. H. (1992). Frail Elders and the Suburbs. *Generations,* Spring, 35-39.

Hartford Insurance Group (1990). *How to modify a home to accommodate the needs of an older adult.* Hartford, CT: Hartford Insurance Group Publications.

Hiatt, L. (1984). Barrier free and prosthetic design: Issues in housing for seniors. *Papers from a symposium on innovations in housing and living arrangements for seniors* (pp. 197-226). Burnaby, British Columbia, Canada: The Gerontology Research Center.

Hiatt, L. (1988a). Technology and dreams of aging. *Perspectives on Aging, 17*(l), 5-8.

Hoglund, David J. (1983). Privacy and independence in housing for the elderly:

The intangible qualities of housing. Washington, DC: National Endowment for the Arts Publications.

Kahana, E. (1974). *A congruence model of person-environment interaction.* Report from conference at Kansas State University. Washington, DC: Gerontological Society.

Lawton, M. P. (1989). Three functions of the residential environment. *Journal of Housing for the Elderly, 5*(1), 35-50.

Lawton, M. P. & Hoover, S. L. (Eds.) (1981). *Community housing choices for older Americans.* New York: Springer.

Luek, O. (1987). *Design for all people.* ASID Report, *8*(2), 8.

Mace, R., Hardie, J., & Pace, J. (1990). Accessible environments: Toward universal design. In W. Preiser, J. Vischer, & E. White (Eds.), *Design Intervention: Toward a More Humane Architecture.* New York: Van Nostrand Reinhold.

McLeister, D. (1989). Are you meeting adaptable housing needs? *Professional Builder,* August.

Mitchelson, W. (1977). *Environmental choice, human behavior and residential satisfaction.* New York: Oxford University Press.

National Center for Health Statistics. (1991). *Prevention Profile.* Hyattsville, MD: Public Health Service.

Null, R. (1989). Universal design for the elderly. *Housing and Society, 16*(3), 77-83.

O'Bryant, S. L. (1983). The subjective value of home to older homeowners. *Journal of Housing for the Elderly, 1*, 29-43.

Palmore, E. B. (1977). Facts on aging: A short quiz. *The Gerontologist, 17,* 315-320.

Pastalan, L. (1988). The rational. *Universal design: Housing for the life span of all people.* Washington, DC: Department of Housing and Urban Development Publication.

Pynoos, J. (1992). Strategies for home modification and repair. *Generations,* Spring, 21-25.

Raschko, B. (1987). Universal Design. *ASID Report, 13*(2), 8-10.

Reizenstein, J. E. (1975). Linking social research and design. *Journal of Architectural Research, 4,* 26-38.

Salmon, F. C. (1963). *Architectural environments for the aging: Restorative medicine in geriatrics.* Springfield, IL: Thomas.

Shapiro, E. & Tate, R. (1988). Who is really at risk of institutionalization? *The Gerontologist, 28*(2), 237-245.

Struyk, R. J. (1977). The housing situations of elderly Americans. *The Gerontologist, 20,* 45-55.

United States Department of Housing and Urban Development (1988). *Universal design: Housing for the life span of all people.* (HUD Publication No. HUD-1155-PA). Washington, DC: Office of Intergovernmental Relations.

Chapter 9

A Mathematical Model
of the Housing Decisions
# of Elderly Homeowners

Peter G. VanderHart

SUMMARY. This article presents a mathematical model that attempts to capture the factors that are most important in determining an elderly homeowner's housing decision. The factors considered include the homeowner's home equity, financial assets, income, housing cost, and psychological attachment to the home. The findings indicate that the various factors may have quite different effects across the varied housing actions that the elderly may take. This suggests that any empirical analysis regarding the home ownership decisions of the elderly needs to distinguish among the different actions that the elderly can take.

INTRODUCTION

This article presents a model that attempts to capture the factors that are most important in determining an elderly homeowner's housing decision. The factors considered include the homeowner's home equity, financial assets, income, housing cost, and psycholog-

Peter G. VanderHart is Assistant Professor of Economics, Department of Economics, Bowling Green State University, Bowling Green, OH 43403-0268.

[Haworth co-indexing entry note]: "A Mathematical Model of the Housing Decisions of Elderly Homeowners." VanderHart, Peter G. Co-published simultaneously in *Journal of Housing for the Elderly* (The Haworth Press, Inc.) Vol. 11, No. 2, 1995, pp. 139-165; and: *Housing Decisions for the Elderly: To Move or Not to Move* (ed: Leon A. Pastalan) The Haworth Press, Inc., 1995, pp. 139-165. Multiple copies of this article/chapter may be purchased from The Haworth Document Delivery Center [1-800-3-HAWORTH; 9:00 a.m. - 5:00 p.m. (EST)].

ical attachment[1] to the home. Although many empirical studies have examined these factors, few have treated them theoretically and none have integrated all of them into a single framework. The theory presented here is similar to earlier work by Artle and Varaiya (1978). It is different because it concentrates only on the aged, explicitly includes preference for home ownership, and treats tenure choice endogenously.

The paper is organized as follows: The next section states the assumptions behind the model and introduces the notation used. A third section explains the derivation of the expression describing the satisfaction received by homeowners who choose to remain in their home. The section after that presents the expressions describing the level of satisfaction that the homeowner could receive if various housing changes are chosen. The fifth section compares the levels of satisfaction and calculates comparative statics. A final section discusses the shortcomings of the model, and summarizes.

ASSUMPTIONS AND NOTATION

We begin by considering an elderly household currently at time 0 with certain time of death T. The household receives instantaneous utility from ordinary consumption and from the amount of owner-occupied housing owned. We assume that the utility function is separable in these two goods, and can be written for any time $t < T$ as

$$(1) \quad U(C_t) + \Gamma_t \cdot \phi_t$$

where C_t is ordinary consumption at time t; Γ_t is the amount of housing owned at time t, (assumed to remain constant unless a housing change is made); $U(\cdot)$ is the utility function on ordinary consumption, (with $U'(\cdot) > 0$ and $U''(\cdot) < 0$); and ϕ_t represents the household's preference for owner-occupied housing, which is assumed to decline through time: $(\phi_t = \phi_0 - \lambda t)$.[2]

The household begins with an endowment of financial assets A_0, and an initial level of home equity H_0, on which there is no mortgage debt. These amounts appreciate at real rates of return r_a and r_h respectively. The household receives a fixed income (I), and pays constant out-of-pocket housing costs (p_o) at each moment. We may then write the household's budget constraint as:

(2) $\dot{H}_t + \dot{A}_t = I - C_t + r_a(A_t) + r_h(H_t) - p_o$

Please note that Γ and H are not the same variable, indicating that amount of housing and its equity are not defined to be equal: They will vary across time due to appreciation of the home equity.

For the time being, we also restrict the household from choosing to live in an owner-occupied home without holding its full value as home equity. The restriction is necessary to prevent the household from choosing $\Gamma_t > 0$ and $H_t = 0$, which would allow the homeowner to sell the home without moving from it. (This restriction will be relaxed in a later section to allow the owner to acquire a mortgage on the home without moving.) We can write the restriction mathematically as:

(3) $H_t / \exp[r_h t] = \Gamma_t \cdot h$

where h is a scaling factor relating the amount of home equity to the corresponding amount of owner-occupied housing. Without loss of generality we assume that h is equal to 1. Please note that (3) does not restrict the household from (simultaneously) changing their levels of H_t and Γ_t at various times, merely that the two terms maintain a (changing) proportional relationship with each other at any given time.

We must also have a restriction on the level of financial assets held, otherwise the household might borrow an infinite amount ($A_t = -\infty$) and consume the proceeds to maximize utility. Requiring terminal assets to be nonnegative ($A_T \geq 0$) would solve the problem, but it would allow the household to hold negative financial assets up to the amount of home equity, and then an instant before death repay the debt by selling the home. This strategy is essentially a costless reverse mortgage, and is not a possibility for most households. We thus require that the household hold nonnegative financial assets at all times:

(4) $A_t \geq 0 \; \forall t$

We also assume that the household has a bequest function, and that the contribution of bequests to lifetime utility depends on the amount of housing and financial assets held at the date of death: $B(A_T, \Gamma_T)$.

Should the household choose to make a housing change, it will bear a psychological cost of moving ξ. To simplify the analysis we assume that ξ is large enough to make multiple housing changes between 0 and T non-optimal.

Given restrictions (2), (3), and (4), the household will maximize its continuous-time discounted utility by choosing C_t and Γ_t over the rest of its lifetime:

$$
(5) \quad \max_{C_t, \Gamma_t} \int_0^T e^{-\delta t} U(C_t) dt + \int_0^T e^{-\delta t} (\Gamma_t \cdot \phi_t) dt -
$$

$$
e^{-\delta t} (\xi \cdot E_t) + e^{-\delta T} B(A_T, \Gamma_T)
$$

$$
\text{s.t.} \quad \dot{H}_t + \dot{A}_t = I - C_t + r_a(A_t) + r_h(H_t) - p_o
$$

$$
H_t / \exp[r_h t] = \Gamma_t
$$

$$
A_t \geq 0 \; \forall t
$$

where δ is the household's rate of time preference, and E_t equals 1 if the household makes a housing change in time t, 0 if not.

UTILITY EXPRESSION
FROM NOT CHANGING HOUSING STATUS

This section derives an expression for the utility that a household receives if it makes no housing changes between times 0 and T, (i.e., $\Gamma_t = \Gamma_0 \; \forall t$). In later sections this will be used as a base case for comparison to various types of housing changes.

For any period that the household does not make an active change in their home equity, we know that $\dot{H}_t = r_h(H_t)$. Using this and equation (2) we may write:

$$
(6) \quad \dot{A}_t = I - C_t + r_a(A_t) - p_o
$$

as the household's budget constraint for times when no equity change occurs. Rearrangement yields an expression for consumption in every such instant:

(7) $C_t = I - p_o + r_a(A_t) - \dot{A}_t$.

For simplicity, it is assumed that the rate of interest is such that (ceteris paribus) consumption will be the same amount for all t. (See Yaari (1964)).[3] Because we have assumed that I and p_o are also constant through time, the amount "dissaved"[4] in any instant, $[r_a(A_t) - \dot{A}_t]$, will also be a constant. This allows us to express the instantaneous change in the level of financial assets as a simple first order differential equation:

(8) $\dot{A}_t = r_a(A_t) - z_n$

where z_n is the constant amount dissaved in any instant. The solution to equation (8) is:

(9) $A_t = A_0 \cdot \exp[r_a t] - \dfrac{z_n}{r_a} \cdot (\exp[r_a t] - 1)$.

Solving this equation for z_n when t = T yields:

(10) $z_n = \dfrac{(A_0 \cdot \exp[r_a T] - A_{TN}) \cdot r_a}{(\exp[r_a T] - 1)}$

where A_{TN} is the terminal asset level. We can then express the household's consumption as:

(11) $C_t = I - p_o + z_n$.

Given this expression for consumption, and knowing that $\Gamma_t = \Gamma_0$ $\forall t$, we can use (5) to write the expression for utility when no housing change is made between 0 and T:

$$(12) \quad \int_0^T e^{-\delta t} U(I - p_o + z_n) dt + \int_0^T e^{-\delta t}(\Gamma_0 \cdot (\phi_0 - \lambda t)) dt +$$

$$e^{-\delta T} B(A_{NT}, \Gamma_0) \quad .$$

Should the household decide to remain in their home until T, it can maximize its utility merely by selecting the optimal level of terminal assets (A_{NT}). The selection of A_{NT} will uniquely define z_n and therefore expression (12).

UTILITY EXPRESSIONS FOR VARIOUS TYPES OF HOUSING CHANGES

In this section we will derive analogous expressions of (12) for several housing changes: (1) Complete home equity liquidation; (2) partial home equity liquidation; (3) an increase in the amount of home equity held; and (4) acquisition of a mortgage. As mentioned above we have assumed that psychological transaction costs are large enough to discourage multiple changes. Although examination of multiple housing changes by the same household is possible, it is not very fruitful. We therefore concentrate on examples involving only one housing change.

Complete Liquidation of Home Equity

The simplest housing change to describe is the complete liquidation of home equity. The homeowner could accomplish this by selling the home and moving to a rental unit, moving in with relatives, entering a nursing home, or switching to a number of other alternative living arrangements. The proceeds of the sale of the home would provide the household with a source of extra consumption, but after the sale the household would no longer enjoy the benefits of home ownership.

Should the household decide to undertake one of the above housing changes, it will do so at some time t_L^*. Therefore, Γ_t will be equal to Γ_0 until time t_L^* and will be equal to zero after:

$$(13) \quad \Gamma_t = \Gamma_0 \qquad 0 < t < t_L^*$$
$$= 0 \qquad t_L^* \leq t < T$$

Similarly, the household will hold the appreciated value of its home equity until t_L^*, and will hold no home equity after:

$$(14) \quad H_t = H_0 \cdot \exp[r_h t] \qquad 0 < t < t_L^*$$
$$= 0 \qquad t_L^* \leq t < T$$

Thus equation (6) will hold in every instant except at the time of liquidation t_L^*. At that time the amount $H_0 \cdot \exp[r_h t_L^*]$ is added to the existing amount of assets. We therefore need separate expressions to describe the amount of dissaving that occurs before and after home equity liquidation. Utilizing the techniques used to derive (10), we find the following expressions for the pre- and post-liquidation dissaving respectively:

$$(15) \quad z_{bL} = \frac{(A_0 \cdot \exp[r_a t_L^*] - A_{Lt*}) \cdot r_a}{(\exp[r_a t_L^*] - 1)} \quad \text{and}$$

$$(16) \quad z'_{aL} = \frac{[(A_{Lt*} + H_0 \cdot \exp[r_h t_L^*])\exp[r_a (T - t_L^*)] - A_{LT})] \cdot r_a}{(\exp[r_a (T - t_L^*)] - 1)}$$

where A_{Lt*} is the level of assets chosen at t_L^* when the household decides to liquidate home equity, and A_{LT} is the terminal level of assets if the household liquidates home equity.

To express the change in consumption after the liquidation, expression (16) must be altered to account for the change in the out-of-pocket cost of housing:

$$(17) \quad z_{aL} = \frac{[(A_{Lt*} + H_0 \cdot \exp[r_h t_L^*])\exp[r_a (T - t_L^*)] - A_{LT}] \cdot r_a}{(\exp[r_a (T - t_L^*)] - 1)} +$$
$$p_0 - p_L$$

where p_L represents the out-of-pocket cost of alternative housing. We are then able to express the utility in the case of complete home equity liquidation at time t_L^* as:

$$(18) \quad \int_0^{t_L^*} e^{-\delta t} U(I - p_o + z_{bL})dt + \int_{t_L^*}^{T} e^{-\delta t} U(I - p_o + z_{aL})dt +$$

$$\int_0^{t_L^*} e^{-\delta t}(\Gamma_0 \cdot (\emptyset_0 - \lambda t))dt - e^{-\delta t}L \cdot \xi + e^{-\delta T}B(A_{LT}, 0)$$

Should the household decide to completely liquidate their home equity at the optimal time t_L^*, it can maximize its utility by selecting the optimal level of terminal assets given liquidation (A_{LT}), and the optimal level of assets at time t_L^* given liquidation (A_{Lt*}). The selection of these two asset levels will uniquely define z_{bL} and z_{aL} and therefore expression (18).

Partial Reduction of Home Equity

The household need not completely liquidate home equity to finance extra consumption. A partial reduction in home equity by moving to an owner-occupied house of lesser value would provide some funds to increase consumption and still allow the household to enjoy some benefits of home ownership.

If the household decides to move to another owner-occupied home of lesser value, it will do so at a time denoted t_P^*. Under these circumstances, Γ_t will be equal to Γ_0 until time t_P^* and will equal some optimal post-move amount of housing (Γ_P) after t_P^*:

$$(19) \quad \Gamma_t = \Gamma_0 \qquad 0 < t < t_P^*$$
$$= \Gamma_P \qquad t_P^* \leq t < T$$

Likewise, the household will hold its original appreciated value of home equity until t_P^*, and will hold an appreciating smaller amount after t_P^*:

(20) $H_t = H_0 \cdot \exp[r_h t]$ $0 < t < t_P^*$

         $= H_P \cdot \exp[r_h(t - t_P^*)]$ $t_P^* \leq t < T$

where H_P is the smaller level of home equity chosen at t_P^*. Recall restriction (3) and note that H_P and Γ_P are governed by the relationship

(21) $H_P/\exp[r_h t_P^*] = \Gamma_P$.

This restriction requires the household to reduce home equity in proportion to its reduction in owner-occupied housing, after appreciation of home equity is accounted for. (A similar condition exists for the case of complete liquidation, but it is trivial since both H_P and Γ_P are equal to 0.) Equation (21) has the effect of not allowing the household to choose high values of Γ_P while simultaneously choosing low values of H_P.

   As in the previous section, equation (6) will hold in every instant except at the time of equity reduction t_P^*. At that time the amount $(H_0 \cdot \exp[r_h t_P^*] - H_P)$ is added to the existing amount of assets. We therefore can find the expressions for the dissaving that occurs before and after a partial reduction in home equity to be:

(22) $z_{bP} = \dfrac{(A_0 \cdot \exp[r_a t_P^*] - A_{Pt^*}) \cdot r_a}{(\exp[r_a t_P^*] - 1)}$ and

(23) $z'_{aP} = \dfrac{\left[(A_{Pt^*} + H_0 \cdot \exp[r_h t_P^*] - H_p)\exp[r_a (T - t_P^*)] - A_{PT}\right] \cdot r_a}{(\exp[r_a(T - t_P^*)] - 1)}$

where A_{Pt^*} is the level of assets chosen at t_P^* when the household decides to partially reduce home equity, and A_{PT} is the terminal level of assets if the household partially reduces home equity.

   To arrive at the expression for the amount of extra consumption derived from partial equity reduction, we must again adjust the post-change dissaving expression to account for the change in out-of-pocket housing costs:

$$(24) \quad z_{aP} = \frac{\left[(A_{P_{t^*}} + H_0 \cdot \exp[r_h t_P^*] - H_p)\exp[r_a (T - t_P^*)] - A_{PT}\right] \cdot r_a}{(\exp[r_a(T - t_P^*)] - 1)}$$
$$+ \; p_o - p_p$$

where pp represents the out-of-pocket housing costs after the household moves to a home of lesser value. We can then express the utility from partial home equity reduction at time t_P^* to be:

$$(25) \quad \int_0^{t_P^*} e^{-\delta t}U(I - p_o + z_{bP})dt + \int_{t_P^*}^{T} e^{-\delta t}U(I - p_o + z_{aP})dt +$$

$$\int_0^{t_P^*} e^{-\delta t}(\Gamma_0 \cdot (\phi_0 - \lambda t))dt + \int_{t_P^*}^{T} e^{-\delta t}(\Gamma_P \cdot (\phi_0 - \lambda t))dt -$$

$$e^{-\delta t_P^*} \cdot \xi + e^{-\delta T}B(A_{PT}, \Gamma_P)$$

If the household decides to partially reduce its home equity at the optimal time t_P^* it will maximize expression (25) by choosing an optimal lower level of housing (Γ_P), (and therefore Hp by expression (21)), an optimal level of assets at time t_P^* given partial reduction ($A_{P_{t^*}}$), and the optimal level of terminal assets given partial reduction (A_{PT}). Choosing these three values uniquely defines expressions (22) and (24) and therefore defines expression (25).

Increase in Home Equity

Of course reducing or liquidating home equity is not the only alternative for current homeowners. Under some circumstances, it may be optimal for a household to increase its home equity by moving to a home of greater value than the current home. A move of this type increases the amount of owner-occupied housing that the homeowner enjoys, but decreases the funds available for consumption expenditures.

We can describe this alternative along the lines of the previous subsections. If a household decides to increase home equity by moving to a home of greater value, it will do so at some time t_I^*. Under these circumstances, Γ_t will be equal to Γ_0 until time t_I^*, and will equal some optimal post-move amount of housing (Γ_I) after t_I^* :

$$(26) \quad \Gamma_t = \Gamma_0 \qquad 0 < t < t_I^*$$
$$ = \Gamma_I \qquad t_I^* \le t < T$$

Analogously to the previous subsection, the amount of home equity held through time can be described by:

$$(27) \quad H_t = H_0 \cdot \exp[r_h t] \qquad 0 < t < t_I^*$$
$$ = H_I \cdot \exp[r_h(t - t_I^*)] \qquad t_I^* \le t < T$$

and H_I and Γ_I will be related to one another by the following equation:

$$(28) \quad H_I/\exp[r_h t_I^*] = \Gamma_I \quad .$$

Equation (6) will be true in every instant except at time t_I^*. At that moment $(H_I - H_0 \cdot \exp[r_h t])$ will be subtracted from the existing amount of assets to finance the increase in home equity. Therefore we may define the dissaving that occurs before and after the increase in home equity to be:

$$(29) \quad z_{bI} = \frac{(A_0 \cdot \exp[r_a t_I^*] - A_{It^*}) \cdot r_a}{(\exp[r_a t_I^*] - 1)} \qquad \text{and}$$

$$(30) \quad z'_{aI} = \frac{[(A_{It^*} + H_0 \cdot \exp[r_h t_I^*] - H_I)\exp[r_a (T - t_I^*)] - A_{IT}] \cdot r_a}{(\exp[r_a(T - t_I^*)] - 1)}$$

where A_{It^*} is the level of assets chosen at t_I^* if the household decides to increase home equity by moving, and A_{IT} is the terminal level of assets when such a move occurs.

Adjusting (30) by including the difference in out-of-pocket costs from the housing change yields:

$$(31) \quad z_{al} = \frac{[(A_{It*} + H_0 \cdot \exp[r_h t_I^*] - H_I)\exp[r_a (T - t_I^*)] - A_{IT}] \cdot r_a}{(\exp[r_a (T - t_I^*)] - 1)}$$
$$+ p_o - p_I$$

where p_I is the out-of-pocket housing cost of the home of greater value. We can then express the utility from increasing home equity by moving at time t_I^* to be:

$$(32) \quad \int_0^{t_I^*} e^{-\delta t} U(I - p_o + z_{bI})dt + \int_{t_I^*}^T e^{-\delta t} U(I - p_o + z_{al})dt +$$

$$\int_0^{t_I^*} e^{-\delta t}(\Gamma_0 \cdot (\phi_0 - \lambda t))dt + \int_{t_I^*}^T e^{-\delta t}(\Gamma_I \cdot (\phi_0 - \lambda t))dt -$$

$$e^{-\delta t_I^*} \cdot \xi + e^{-\delta T} B(A_{IT}, \Gamma_I)$$

If the household chooses to increase its home equity by moving to another home at time t_I^*, it will do so by choosing an optimal greater level of housing (Γ_I), an optimal level of assets at time t_I^* (A_{It*}), and an optimal level of terminal assets given the increase in home equity (A_{IT}). Choosing these values uniquely defines expression (32) via expressions (28), (29) and (31).

Acquisition of a Mortgage

The final housing change explored in this chapter is the acquisition of a new mortgage on the presently occupied home. Mortgaging one's home may be an attractive way of utilizing home equity because it allows a household to utilize the value of the home to finance extra consumption without incurring the psychological and transaction costs of moving. However, acquiring a new mortgage also has some disadvantages: High finance charges from the mortgage will reduce the supplemental consumption from the proceeds of the loan; and the level of home equity held by the household will gradually increase, rather than decrease, as the mortgage is paid off.

As with the baseline (no change) alternative described above, the amount of housing held by a homeowner who chooses to acquire a mortgage will remain constant between 0 and T: ($\Gamma_t = \Gamma_0 \, \forall t$). However, home equity will take a more complicated path, and it will no longer conform to equation (3). It will increase at rate r_h, just as it does in the other alternatives, until time t_M^*, the date that the household acquires a new mortgage. At t_M^*, home equity will fall by the amount of home equity that is mortgaged, $k \cdot (H_0 \cdot \exp[r_h t_M^*])$, where k is the percentage of home equity at time t_M^* that is mortgaged. After t_M^*, home equity will increase by the amount of appreciation on the entire value of home equity plus the amount of principle that is paid off in any instant. The path is summarized in the following equations:

$$(33) \quad H_t = H_0 \cdot \exp[r_h t] \qquad 0 < t < t_M^*$$

$$= H_0 \cdot \exp[r_h t] - M_t \qquad t_M^* \leq t < T$$

where M_t is the amount of mortgage principle owed at time t and can be expressed by:

$$(34) \quad M_t = \left[k \cdot H_0 \cdot \exp[r_h t_M^*]\right] \cdot$$

$$\left[\exp[r_m(t - t_M^*)] - \frac{\exp[r_m(T_M - t_M^*)] \cdot (\exp[r_m(t - t_M^*)] - 1)}{\exp[r_m(T_M - t_M^*)] - 1}\right]$$

where T_M denotes the date that the mortgage is paid off, which may be before or after the date of death T.

As in the previous subsections, equation (6) will hold at every instant except at t_M^*, when the amount $(k \cdot H_0 \cdot \exp[r_h t_M^*])$ is added to the existing level of assets. We also assume that acquiring the mortgage costs a one-time fixed amount C. The amount of dissaving before and after the acquisition of the mortgage can then be written as follows:

$$(35) \quad z_{bM} = \frac{(A_0 \cdot \exp[r_a t_M^*] - A_{Mt^*}) \cdot r_a}{(\exp[r_a \, t_M^*] - 1)} \qquad \text{and}$$

$$(36) \quad z'_{aM} = \frac{\left[(A_{Mt^*} + kH_0 \exp[r_h t_M^*] - C)\exp[r_a (T - t_M^*)] - A_{MT}\right] \cdot r_a}{(\exp[r_a (T - t_M^*)] - 1)}$$

where A_{Mt^*} is the optimal asset level at time t_M^* if a new mortgage is acquired, and A_{MT} is the optimal level of assets at the date of death should a new mortgage be obtained.

To adjust (36) to represent consumption after the mortgage is acquired, we note that p_0 will still be paid, in addition to mortgage payment p_M. Therefore consumption after the mortgage is acquired can be expressed by:

$$(37) \quad z_{aM} = \frac{\left[(A_{Mt^*} + kH_0 \exp[r_h t_M^*] - C)\exp[r_a (T - t_M^*)] - A_{MT}\right] \cdot r_a}{(\exp[r_a (T - t_M^*)] - 1)}$$
$$- p_M \,.$$

Solving the differential equation that describes the movement of remaining mortgage principal yields the following equation for p_M:

$$(38) \quad p_M = \frac{\left[k \cdot H_0 \cdot \exp[r_h t_M^*] \cdot \exp[r_m(T_M - t_M^*)] \cdot r_m\right]}{(\exp[r_m (T_M - t_M^*)] - 1} \,.$$

We therefore can write the expression for the utility of a household who decides to acquire a new mortgage at time t_M^* as:

$$(39) \quad \int_0^{t_M^*} e^{-\delta t}U(I - p_0 + z_{bM})dt + \int_{t_M^*}^{T} e^{-\delta t}U(I - p_0 + z_{aM})dt +$$

$$\int_0^{T} e^{-\delta t}(\Gamma_0 \cdot (\emptyset_0 - \lambda t))dt + e^{-\delta T}B(A_{MT} - M_T, \Gamma_0)$$

where M_T is the remaining mortgage principal owed at the time of death, and is defined by expression (34). We assume that it appears in the bequest function as being subtracted from the terminal level of assets.

Should the household choose to acquire a mortgage at the optimal choice of time t_M^*, it will maximize expression (39) by choosing A_{Mt^*}, the level of financial assets at t_M^*; A_{MT}, the level of financial assets at the time of death; and M_T, the amount of outstanding mortgage principle at the time of death. The household's choice of M_T, (along with market-defined r_m and T_M) defines k via equation (34). Using k, A_{Mt^*}, and A_{MT}, we can find (35) and (37) and thus uniquely define expression (39).

No doubt the reader has noticed that expressions (18), (25), (32), and (39) share a similar form and are derived in a similar manner. Indeed one could think of these expressions as being particular examples of a more general expression that allows the homeowner to choose over all housing alternatives (and all Γ_t) in any period to maximize utility. The separate expressions are explicitly stated because in later sections each will be used to calculate comparative statics that vary across alternatives.

It may be possible to describe other sorts of housing changes, such as taking other people into the home to share expenses, moving from a smaller to a larger home by acquiring a mortgage on the new home, or allowing home maintenance to go undone, thereby saving money that could be used for consumption. A particularly inviting extension would be to allow households to move to areas where a given amount of home equity buys a greater amount of owner-occupied housing. However for the time being we will limit ourselves to the previously mentioned housing changes as the available alternatives for elderly homeowners.

THE UTILITY GAIN FROM HOUSING CHANGES AND COMPARATIVE STATICS

In the previous section we derived expressions for the utility that a household receives under different housing changes. In this section we examine the conditions under which these changes will actually occur, and the factors that affect the decision to make the changes. We begin by examining expressions that describe the gain in utility from making each of the previously described housing changes. Then by using partial differentiation, we derive comparative statics.

The Gain from Liquidation

An expression for the gain from home equity liquidation can be found by subtracting expression (12) from expression (18). By splitting the integral in expression (12) and recombining terms we find:

$$(40) \quad \int_0^{t_L^*} e^{-\delta t} \left[U(I - p_o + z_{bL}) - U(I - p_o + z_n) \right] dt + \int_{t_L^*}^{T} e^{-\delta t}$$

$$\left[U(I - p_o + z_{aL}) - U(I - p_o + z_n) \right] dt - \int_{t_L^*}^{T} e^{-\delta t}(\Gamma_0 \cdot (\emptyset_0 - \lambda t))$$

$$dt - e^{-\delta t_L^*} \cdot \xi + e^{-\delta T}[B(A_{LT}, 0) - B(A_{NT}, \Gamma_0)] \quad .$$

Evaluating the integrals and taking second order Taylor approximations around the z terms gives us:

$$(41) \quad G_L = \frac{[1 - \exp(-\delta t_L^*)]}{\delta} \left[(z_{bL} - z_n) \cdot U'(I - p_o) + \frac{(z_{bL})^2 - (z_n)^2}{2} \cdot U''(I - p_o) \right] +$$

$$\frac{[\exp(-\delta t_L^*) - \exp(-\delta T)]}{\delta} \cdot \left[(z_{aL} - z_n) \cdot U'(I - p_o) + \frac{(z_{aL})^2 - (z_n)^2}{2} \cdot U''(I - p_o) \right] -$$

$$\frac{\Gamma_0}{\delta} [\exp(-\delta t_L^*) \cdot [\emptyset_0 - \lambda t_L^* - \lambda/\delta] - \exp(-\delta T) \cdot [\emptyset_0 - \lambda T - \lambda/\delta]] -$$

$$\xi [\exp(-\delta t_L^*)] + e^{-\delta T}[B(A_{LT}, 0) - B(A_{NT}, \Gamma_0)] \quad .$$

In expression (41), the first line represents the utility gain between 0 and t_L^* from the extra consumption made possible by the future home equity liquidation. The second line represents the utility gain between t_L^* and T from the extra consumption after home equity is liquidated. The third line represents the forgone utility from not owning any owner-occupied housing from t_L^* to T; and the last line is the loss in utility due to the housing change, and the difference in utility from bequests.

The expression for G_L may be positive or negative depending on the values of the underlying parameters. It will attain its greatest value at the optimal value t_L^*, and if $G_L \mid t_L^* > 0$, the household may liquidate home equity at that time.

Comparative Statics for Liquidation

At this point expression (41) remains general in the sense that the z terms need not be positive (i.e., the household can either be saving or dissaving between 0 and T). However, to evaluate the signs of the comparative statics below we assume $z_{bL}, z_{aL} > z_n > 0$; that is, the elderly do dissave out of financial assets and they dissave more if they liquidate home equity.

Because t_L^*, A_{Lt*}, A_{NT}, and A_{LT} are all defined as choice variables, the envelope theorem applies to them when performing comparative statics. This is a tremendous help when trying to sign the derivatives. Differentiating expression (41) with respect to certain variables yields a number of interesting relationships:

$\dfrac{\partial G_L}{\partial H_0} > 0$ A higher initial value of home equity means that the home will be worth more when sold, and thus provide greater increased consumption.

$\dfrac{\partial G_L}{\partial A_0} < 0$ The utility from an extra unit of initial financial assets is greater when the household does not choose to liquidate home equity. An extra amount of assets will increase consumption in both the liquidation and no liquidation cases, but it will be more valuable in utility terms in the no liquidation case due to diminishing marginal utility. Intuitively, greater financial wealth makes equity liquidation less necessary to sustain consumption.

$\dfrac{\partial G_L}{\partial I} < 0$ The greater a household's income the less need they have to supplement it with liquidated home equity.

$\dfrac{\partial G_L}{\partial p_o} > 0$ The higher the cost of owner-occupied housing, the more attractive alternative housing arrangements are.

$\dfrac{\partial G_L}{\partial p_L} < 0$ The higher the cost of alternative housing, the less attractive home equity liquidation.

$\dfrac{\partial G_L}{\partial \emptyset_0} < 0$ The greater the initial utility from each unit of owner-occupied housing owned, the less the gain one will receive from leaving it.

$\dfrac{\partial G_L}{\partial \lambda} > 0$ The faster the deterioration in a household's preference for home ownership, the greater the gain in utility from equity liquidation.

To the extent that these relationships represent increases or decreases in the gain from liquidating home equity, they also represent increases or decreases in a household's propensity to liquidate home equity by leaving the current home for other accommodations. They therefore represent a set of testable hypotheses.

The Gain from Partial Reduction

The expression for the utility gain from partial home equity reduction can be found using the same method used above. First we subtract expression (12) from (25). We then split the integrals of (12) and rearrange terms. After evaluating the integrals, performing second order Taylor approximations and simplifying, we find the utility gain from partial home equity liquidation to be:

$$(42) \quad G_p = \frac{[1 - \exp(-\delta t_p^*)]}{\delta}$$

$$\left[(z_{bP} - z_n) \cdot U'(I - p_o) + \frac{(z_{bP})^2 - (z_n)^2}{2} \cdot U''(I - p_o) \right] +$$

$$\frac{[\exp(-\delta t_p^*) - \exp(-\delta T)]}{\delta} \cdot$$

$$\left[(z_{aP} - z_n) \cdot U'(I - p_o) + \frac{(z_{aP})^2 - (z_n)^2}{2} \cdot U''(I - p_o) \right] -$$

$$\frac{\Gamma_0 - \Gamma_P}{\delta} \cdot$$

$$\left[\exp(-\delta t_P^*) \cdot [\emptyset_0 - \lambda t_P^* - \lambda/\delta] - \exp(-\delta T) \cdot [\emptyset_0 - \lambda T - \lambda/\delta] \right] -$$

$$\xi \, [\exp(-\delta t_P^*)] + e^{-\delta T}[B(A_{PT}, \Gamma_P) - B(A_{NT}, \Gamma_0)] \; .$$

Expression (42) is very similar to its predecessor describing complete liquidation, and has the same interpretation. Note the difference in the third line, which describes the lost utility from not owning the original amount of housing. In (42) this line is a smaller negative value due to the fact that some housing is still owned. The expression also differs from (41) in that the z terms are a different value, and that the utility from bequests is different.

As in the case of complete liquidation, the expression for G_P may be positive or negative. The household will choose to partially reduce its home equity only if G_P is greater than 0 at time t_P^*.

Comparative Statics for Partial Reduction

The comparative statics for partial home equity reduction are completely analogous to those found in section 5.2, (with the exception that ∂p_P should replace ∂p_L), so for the sake of brevity they will not be repeated.

The Gain from an Increase in Home Equity

We find the expression for the gain in utility from an increase in home equity in the same way as before, this time by subtracting expression (12) from (32). Performing the mathematical operations described earlier yields the following expression:

$$(43) \quad G_I = \frac{[1 - \exp(-\delta t_I^*)]}{\delta}$$

$$\left[(z_{bI} - z_n) \cdot U'(I - p_o) + \frac{(z_{bI})^2 - (z_n)^2}{2} \cdot U''(I - p_o) \right] +$$

$$\frac{[\exp(-\delta t_I^*) - \exp(-\delta T)]}{\delta} \; .$$

$$\left[(z_{aI} - z_n) \cdot U'(I - p_o) + \frac{(z_{aI})^2 - (z_n)^2}{2} \cdot U''(I - p_o) \right] -$$

$$\frac{\Gamma_0 - \Gamma_I}{\delta} \cdot$$

$$\left[\exp(- \delta t_I^*) \cdot [\phi_0 - \lambda t_I^* - \lambda/\delta] - \exp(- \delta T) \cdot [\phi_0 - \lambda T - \lambda/\delta] \right] -$$

$$\xi \, [\exp(- \delta t_I^*)] + e^{- \delta T}[B(A_{IT}, \Gamma_I) - B(A_{NT}, \Gamma_0)]$$

Although this expression takes the same form as (41) and (42), it is different in significant ways. First, we now will assume that households who buy houses having more equity will dissave out of financial assets less than those who don't. Mathematically, z_{bI} and z_{aI} will be less than z_n. This means that the expressions for the difference in utility from the change in consumption will now be negative, rather than positive as in expressions (41) and (42). Also, since Γ_I, is greater than Γ_0, the expression for change in utility from housing (the fourth line in (42)) will now be positive. These changes will cause a number of differences in the comparative statics described presently.

Comparative Statics for Increase in Home Equity

To evaluate the signs of the following expressions, we assume that $z_n > z_{bI}$, and $z_{aI} > 0$; that is, that the elderly dissave out of financial assets even when they purchase a more expensive home, but that they dissave less than if no housing change is made. Differentiating expression (43) with respect to the variables of interest yields the following:

$\dfrac{\partial G_I}{\partial H_0} > 0$ This result is somewhat counterintuitive. It occurs because a higher level of initial home equity makes it easier to buy a home of even larger equity without reducing the financial assets that will provide increased consumption.

$\dfrac{\partial G_I}{\partial A_0} > 0$ An extra amount of assets will increase consumption in both the equity increase and the no change cases, but it will be more valuable in utility terms in the equity increase case due to diminishing marginal utility. Intuitively, greater financial wealth makes an equity increase easier.

$\dfrac{\partial G_I}{\partial I} > 0$ The greater a household's income the easier it is to increase home equity without reducing consumption.

$\dfrac{\partial G_I}{\partial p_0} \begin{smallmatrix} > \\ < \end{smallmatrix} 0?$ Intuition would tell us that original housing that is more expensive would cause homeowners to find alternative housing arrangements. This is true, but the higher initial housing costs also make it more difficult for a household to afford a home with higher equity. It is impossible to determine which factor dominates.

$\dfrac{\partial G_I}{\partial p_I} < 0$ The higher the cost of the home with higher home equity, the less attractive the option seems.

$\dfrac{\partial G_I}{\partial \emptyset_0} > 0$ The greater the initial utility from each unit of owner-occupied housing, the more the household has to gain by increasing the amount of housing.

$\dfrac{\partial G_I}{\partial \lambda} < 0$ The faster the deterioration in a household's preference for home ownership, the smaller the gain in utility from increasing the amount of housing owned.

These relationships provide us with additional testable hypotheses.

The Gain from Mortgage Acquisition

To derive the expression describing the utility gain from acquiring a new mortgage, we first subtract expression (12) from (39). After splitting the integral in (12), evaluating all the integrals, and performing a second order Taylor approximation around the z terms, we find the following:

$$(44) \quad G_M = \frac{[1 - \exp(-\delta t_M^*)]}{\delta}$$

$$\left[(z_{bM} - z_n) \cdot U'(I - p_o) + \frac{(z_{bM})^2 - (z_n)^2}{2} \cdot U''(I - p_o) \right] +$$

$$\frac{[\exp(-\delta t_M^*) - \exp(-\delta T)]}{\delta} \cdot$$

$$\left[(z_{aM} - z_n) \cdot U'(I - p_o) + \frac{(z_{aM})^2 - (z_n)^2}{2} \cdot U''(I - p_o) \right] +$$

$$e^{-\delta T}[B(A_{MT} - M_T, \Gamma_0) - B(A_{NT}, \Gamma_0)] \quad .$$

This expression differs from the earlier expressions in that there are no terms describing the psychological transaction cost or the difference in utility from owning a different amount of housing. Because the household continues to live in the same home, there is no utility cost or change in housing from moving. The financial transaction cost from acquiring a mortgage, C, is embodied in z_{aM}.

As with the preceding utility gain expressions, (44) may be either positive or negative. It will attain its greatest value at an optimal time t_M^*. If the expression is positive at that time then the household may acquire a new mortgage.

Comparative Statics for Mortgage Acquisition

For the evaluation of these expressions we adopt similar assumptions to those used in subsections 5.2 and 5.4. Specifically, we assume that z_{bM} and z_{aM} are greater than z_n; that is, that the household will dissave at a greater rate if it chooses to acquire a new mortgage. Taking partial derivatives of (44) with respect to the variables of interest yields the following:

$\dfrac{\partial G_M}{\partial H_0} > 0$ A higher initial value of home equity means that a greater amount of home equity can be mortgaged, thus providing greater increased consumption.

$\dfrac{\partial G_M}{\partial A_0} < 0$ An extra amount of assets will increase consumption in both the mortgage acquisition and no change cases, but it will be more valuable in utility terms in the no change case due to diminishing marginal utility. Intuitively, greater financial wealth makes acquiring a new mortgage less necessary to sustain consumption.

$\dfrac{\partial G_M}{\partial I} < 0$ The greater a household's income the less need they have to supplement it with proceeds from a mortgage.

$\dfrac{\partial G_M}{\partial p_o} > 0$ The higher the cost of owner-occupied housing, the more valuable the proceeds from a mortgage.

$\dfrac{\partial G_M}{\partial p_m} < 0$ The higher the cost of financing the mortgage, the less attractive this alternative will be.

$\dfrac{\partial G_M}{\partial \phi_0} = 0$ Because acquiring a new mortgage does not change the amount of housing occupied, any change in the amount that it is enjoyed will have no effect on the gain from acquiring a mortgage.

$\dfrac{\partial G_M}{\partial \lambda} = 0$ As with ϕ_0, a change in the rate of deterioration of the preference for housing will have no effect on the gain in utility from mortgage acquisition.

These comparative statics are added to the testable hypotheses derived in the previous sections.

SHORTCOMINGS OF THE MODEL

This model, as it stands, is flawed in a number of ways. Most noticeably, it lacks any randomness with respect to utility from home ownership, income, expenses, and time of death. The uncertainty created by unexpected variations of such factors almost certainly has an effect on homeowners' decisions. However, including stochastic elements in the present framework is very burdensome and does not yield tractable results.

The model also suffers from a rather simple treatment of the utility from housing. Specifically, it does not differentiate the utility from various non-owning housing arrangements from one another, (it merely defines $\emptyset_t$ as the difference in utility between owner-occupied and all other types of housing), and assumes a linear utility function for owner-occupied housing. However, enhancing the model to treat these problems would cause the model to be even more cumbersome and would add little to the understanding of the behavior we wish to explore.

CONCLUSIONS

To the extent that the results of the previous sections represent changes in the utility gain from various housing changes, they will also represent changes in the propensity of homeowners to choose the various alternatives. By observing the actions of homeowners we can estimate the effect of the various factors on the homeowners' propensity to choose the alternatives and thus the utility gain they receive. The results are therefore empirically testable.

The theoretic results of this article are summarized in Table 1, which describes the effect of various factors on the gain from the housing changes. These results are fairly simple and for the most part are intuitive. As the reader can see, the factors have differing effects across the various housing changes. This suggests that any empirical analysis regarding the home ownership decisions of the elderly needs to distinguish among the different actions that the elderly can take, and allow for the fact that any one factor may have different effects on the propensity to the various actions.

Past empirical studies have not been consistent with the theoretic implications of the model. Specifically, several past analyses (Venti and Wise (1989), Feinstein and McFadden (1987), Stahl (1989)) have focused merely on mobility when analyzing the housing decisions of the elderly. This tends to group several types of housing changes together (buying a larger home, buying a smaller home, moving to a rental unit, moving to a dependent living arrangement) when the results described in this paper suggest that a disaggregated approach is more appropriate. Concentrating only on mobility also ignores actions such as acquiring a mortgage that change home equity without a move.

Other articles, while distinguishing among some types of housing actions, still group some moves together when it is not appropriate. VanderHart (1993) merely distinguishes equity reducing actions

TABLE 1. Summary of Theoretic Results Change in Utility Gain from Housing Changes for Increases in Various Factors

Factor	Utility Gain From		
	Equity Reduction/ Liquidation	Equity Increase	Mortgage Acquisition
Home Equity	Increase	Increase	Increase
Financial Assets	Decrease	Increase	Decrease
Income	Decrease	Increase	Decrease
Current Housing Costs	Increase	?	Increase
Alternative Housing Costs	Decrease	Decrease	Decrease
Preference for Home Ownership	Decrease	Increase	0
Reduction in Preference for Ownership	Increase	Decrease	0

from all other actions, and Merrill (1984) combines own-to-own transitions when some are equity-reducing and some are equity-increasing. Both of these analyses violate the theoretical results described above, which point out that certain factors have quite different effects on different types of housing changes.

An important result of this theoretical analysis is that housing wealth and financial wealth will have opposite effects on the utility gains from equity reduction. This suggests that a well-formulated study should disaggregate the two forms of wealth when examining their effect on housing actions. Several previous authors (Venti and Wise (1989), Feinstein and McFadden (1987)) have not done so, and merely combine financial assets and home equity into a single measure of wealth. Their mixed findings may be a result of combining two factors that have very opposite effects.

An important question that remains essentially unanswered by the literature is that of which of the factors are more important. Not only is there a question about which financial factors are most important, but it remains unclear whether financial factors or demographic factors dominate the decision. The present mathematical treatment offers little guidance because one must assume particular values for the underlying parameters of the model. Only a few empirical studies (Merrill (1984) and VanderHart (1993)) have used both demographic and economic variables in their analyses, and they suffer from a variety of statistical shortcomings. The topic remains fertile for both theoretic and empirical research.

ENDNOTES

1. I assume that the psychological attachment to the home is a function of marital status, number of children, age, health status, and other demographic characteristics of household members. These factors are not explicitly included in the model, but rather enter implicitly via (ϕ_t).

2. The parameter ϕ_t should be thought of as the difference between the utility of living in owner-occupied housing and the utility from living in non-owner-occupied housing.

3. This essentially means that $r_a = \delta$. For consumption to be a constant when a home equity change takes place, we need $r_h = r_a = \delta$ or another r_h and r_a such that the return on the entire wealth portfolio equals δ. Relaxing this assumption would "tilt" consumption by causing the optimal consumption path to grow if $r_a > \delta$, and to fall if $r_a < \delta$. In either case the theoretical results of the chapter should hold, but the complexity of their derivation would be unnecessarily high.

4. By "dissaved" I mean that households will consume some amount out of their assets and proceeds from assets. Please note that a household could dissave a positive amount and still have assets growing as long as it dissaved less than $r_a(A_t)$ in any instant. In other words, the level of assets will change by the amount it appreciates minus the amount dissaved.

REFERENCES

Artle, Roland, and Varaiya, Pravin, "Life Cycle Consumption and Homeownership," *Journal of Economic Theory* 18, pp. 38-58, 1978.

Feinstein, Jonathan, and McFadden, Daniel, "The Dynamics of Housing Demand by the Elderly: Wealth, Cash Flow, and Demographic Effects," NBER Working Paper #2471, 1987.

Merrill, Sally, "Home Equity and the Elderly," in *Retirement and Economic Behavior*, in H. Aaron and G. Burtless (eds.), Brookings Institution, 1984.

Stahl, Konrad, "Housing Patterns and Mobility of the Aged: The United States and West Germany," in *The Economics of Aging*, in D. Wise (ed.), University of Chicago Press, 1989.

VanderHart, Peter, "A Binomial Probit Analysis of the Home Equity Decisions of Elderly Homeowners," *Research on Aging* 15, pp. 299-323, 1993.

Venti, Steven, and Wise, David, "Aging, Moving, and Housing Wealth," in *The Economics of Aging*, D. Wise (ed.), University of Chicago Press, 1989.

Yaari, Menahem, "On the Consumer's Lifetime Allocation Process," *International Economic Review* 5, pp. 304-317, 1964.

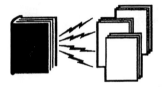

Haworth
DOCUMENT DELIVERY
SERVICE

This new service provides a single-article order form for any article from a Haworth journal.

- *Time Saving:* No running around from library to library to find a specific article.
- *Cost Effective:* All costs are kept down to a minimum.
- *Fast Delivery:* Choose from several options, including same-day FAX.
- *No Copyright Hassles:* You will be supplied by the original publisher.
- *Easy Payment:* Choose from several easy payment methods.

Open Accounts Welcome for...
- Library Interlibrary Loan Departments
- Library Network/Consortia Wishing to Provide Single-Article Services
- Indexing/Abstracting Services with Single Article Provision Services
- Document Provision Brokers and Freelance Information Service Providers

MAIL or *FAX* THIS ENTIRE ORDER FORM TO:

Haworth Document Delivery Service
The Haworth Press, Inc.
10 Alice Street
Binghamton, NY 13904-1580

or FAX: (607) 722-6362
or CALL: 1-800-3-HAWORTH
(1-800-342-9678; 9am-5pm EST)

PLEASE SEND ME PHOTOCOPIES OF THE FOLLOWING SINGLE ARTICLES:
1) Journal Title: _____
   Vol/Issue/Year:_____Starting & Ending Pages:_____
Article Title:_____

2) Journal Title: _____
   Vol/Issue/Year:_____Starting & Ending Pages:_____
Article Title:_____

3) Journal Title: _____
   Vol/Issue/Year:_____Starting & Ending Pages:_____
Article Title:_____

4) Journal Title: _____
   Vol/Issue/Year:_____Starting & Ending Pages:_____
Article Title:_____

(See other side for Costs and Payment Information)

COSTS: Please figure your cost to order quality copies of an article.

1. Set-up charge per article: $8.00
   ($8.00 × number of separate articles)   _____

2. Photocopying charge for each article:

   1-10 pages: $1.00   _____

   11-19 pages: $3.00   _____

   20-29 pages: $5.00   _____

   30+ pages: $2.00/10 pages   _____

3. Flexicover (optional): $2.00/article   _____

4. Postage & Handling: US: $1.00 for the first article/
   $.50 each additional article   _____

   Federal Express: $25.00   _____

   Outside US: $2.00 for first article/
   $.50 each additional article_____

5. Same-day FAX service: $.35 per page   _____

   GRAND TOTAL: _____

METHOD OF PAYMENT: (please check one)

❑ Check enclosed   ❑ Please ship and bill. PO # _____
(sorry we can ship and bill to bookstores only! All others must pre-pay)

❑ Charge to my credit card: ❑ Visa; ❑ MasterCard; ❑ American Express;

Account Number:_____ Expiration date:_____

Signature: *X*_____

Name: _____ Institution: _____

Address: _____

_____

City: _____ State:_____ Zip:_____

Phone Number: _____ FAX Number: _____

MAIL or *FAX* THIS ENTIRE ORDER FORM TO:

Haworth Document Delivery Service	**or FAX:** (607) 722-6362
The Haworth Press, Inc.	**or CALL:** 1-800-3-HAWORTH
10 Alice Street	(1-800-342-9678; 9am-5pm EST)
Binghamton, NY 13904-1580	